UA 50   WEBSKIR BU

D1352023

THE HEALING ENVIRONMENT

Without and within

Edited by

Deborah Kirklin & Ruth Richardson

Royal College of Physicians of London

Publisher's acknowledgement

The Royal College of Physicians acknowledges the generous sponsorship of this book by The Jerwood Foundation, in association with Arts Council England

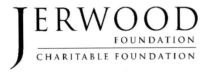

FOUNDATION

CHARITABLE FOUNDATION

Arts Council England is the national development agency for the arts. As part of its work it is committed to supporting and promoting arts-based health initiatives

Front cover

The cover features Anam Cara by the artist Michael Petrone, who is one of the contributors to this book.

Royal College of Physicians of London
11 St Andrew's Place, London NW1 4LE

Registered Charity No. 210508

Copyright © 2003 Royal College of Physicians of London

ISBN 1 86016 191 X

Design and page layout by Merriton Sharp, London
Typeset by Danset Graphics, Telford
Printed in Great Britain by Sarum ColourView, Salisbury

Contents

Contributors

The contributors to this book are active in pioneering the use of the arts and humanities to enhance human health and well-being. A number of them are associated with the Centre for Medical Humanities based in the Department of Primary Care and Population Sciences at the Royal Free and University College Medical School (hereafter referred to as the Centre for Medical Humanities).

Michael Anderson, an artist, is manager of the Mind Arts Project in Stockport.

Kenneth Calman, a physician, is Vice Chancellor and Warden of the University of Durham, and a former Chief Medical Officer.

Lara Dose, a creative thinker, is Director of the National Network for the Arts in Health.

Jane Duncan, an artist, is a Research Assistant and Leverhulme Artist in Residence at the Centre for Medical Humanities.

Claire Elliott, a general practitioner, is a Teaching Fellow in Medical Humanities at the Centre for Medical Humanities.

John Fox, a certified poetry therapist, is President of the National Association for Poetry Therapy.

Roger Higgs, a general practitioner, is Professor of General Practice at Guy's, King's and St Thomas' School of Medicine.

Ghislaine Kenyon, an art historian, is Head of Learning at Somerset House.

Deborah Kirklin, a general practitioner, is the Pfizer Senior Lecturer in Medical Humanities, and Director of the Centre for Medical Humanities.

Susan Loppert, an art historian, is the Director of Chelsea and Westminster Hospital Arts.

Michele Petrone, an artist, is an Honorary Lecturer in Medical Humanities at the Centre for Medical Humanities, and Director of the MAP Foundation.

Ruth Richardson, an interdisciplinary historian, is a Research Associate at the Centre for Medical Humanities.

Michael Rowe, a sociologist, is an Associate Clinical Professor in the Department of Psychiatry at Yale School of Medicine.

Rosalia Staricoff, a neuroscientist, is Director of the Research Project at Chelsea and Westminster Hospital Arts.

John Wells-Thorpe, an architect, is former president of the Commonwealth Association of Architects, and founding chairman of South Downs National Health Service Trust.

A message from the President of the Royal College of Physicians

Concern about the physical and social environments in which medicine is practised – and in which the healing process occurs – is not new. Historically, society's approach has been at best philanthropic and at worst paternalistic; a culture of health care in which staff and, in particular, patients were expected to be passive recipients.

Thankfully, that is now changing. Not only are we beginning to understand and pay more heed to the context in which patients experience illness and care but, more importantly, we are engaging and involving staff and patients in shaping this environment.

From architecture through art therapies to medical humanities, this book looks at how meaningful partnerships between patients, artists, clinicians, architects and managers can make a contribution of immeasurable importance to the development and practice of patient-centred care.

It is invaluable because it provides a clear conceptual framework for understanding the healing environment and, moreover, because it gives examples of good practice and of the exciting possibilities that such interdisciplinary partnerships can generate.

The evidence put forward is compelling and convincing. It is, therefore, a book that will both advance the debate and influence practice. The College is proud to commend it to you.

The College is particularly pleased to be associated with the Jerwood Foundation and Arts Council England in bringing this book to publication.

PROFESSOR CAROL BLACK
President, Royal College of Physicians
October 2003

Statement by the Chairman of the Jerwood Foundation

The arts, education and medicine are at the forefront of all that we do. The publication of *The Healing Environment* embraces all three of these passions.

In recent years the Foundation has sponsored art, music, opera and drama in prisons. I believe there is common ground in this book with our purpose of educating, healing and enlightening through the arts.

We are very pleased, and are rewarded ourselves, to be the principal sponsor of this ground-breaking, learned and stimulating publication by the Royal College of Physicians.

ALAN GRIEVE
Chairman, The Jerwood Foundation
October 2003

Editors' preface

This book is written for all those affected by illness – those who are ill, and those who care.

People who are ill, and the people whose professional task it is to care for them, face challenges in reconciling the medical and social worlds they find themselves simultaneously inhabiting. Our contributors describe how architecture, public art, arts in health, art therapies, community arts, medical humanities and clinical medicine are beginning to work together to help improve the environments in which illness and caring are experienced. We hope readers will be inspired and encouraged by the breadth and variety of work taking place across this developing field.

This volume closes with ideas for further reading drawn from the contributors' suggestions.

DEBORAH KIRKLIN & RUTH RICHARDSON
Centre for Medical Humanities,
Royal Free and University College Medical School, London.

Acknowledgements

Our first thanks must go to all of the contributors who have worked so hard to make this beautiful book possible, and to Andrew Lamb, Diana Beaven, Peter Watkins and Dorothy Sharp at the Royal College of Physicians for their expertise, support and enthusiasm in bringing this volume to press.

The national conference, 'The healing environment: without and within', was held at the National Gallery, London, in March 2001. It acted as a stimulus for a number of chapters, and was supported by educational grants from Pfizer Limited, the Nuffield Trust and the Cancer Research Campaign (now Cancer Research UK).

We are indebted to our colleagues in the Centre for Medical Humanities for their help throughout this project, and in particular to Heather Mitchell for her outstanding administration of everything the Centre does.

Dedication

We dedicate this book to all those who are using their creativity to help build a healing environment for us all,

and to our children, Joshie, Hannah, Sophie, Josh and Charlotte.

DK
RR

Foreword

My job, as Director of the National Network for the Arts in Health, takes me all over the country. I meet many people who either work with, or benefit from, the use of the arts in health. On a train to the south coast recently, a perfect stranger told me his son was recovering from a brain tumour. He and his wife had found, in a hospital waiting room, a copy of a comic strip that explained cancer and its treatment. It was so helpful and easy to understand that they shared it not only with their young son, but also with family and friends. 'It explained everything to everyone better than we could.' The man went on to describe in detail the hospital's art trail, a suggested route around the hospital following key pieces of art. He smiled as he recalled the clown doctors that would visit the ward. 'It might sound strange,' he said, 'to be laughing at a time like that, but it really helped.' There were also performances at the hospital for the patients, visitors and staff. Despite being completely paralysed following his surgery, the man's son always insisted on attending. It was through playing with finger puppets that he regained the ability to speak. The man finished his story by saying, 'I just don't understand why there isn't more of it.'

As this story illustrates, the contemporary arts in health field is about far more than paintings on walls and decorating medical facilities. This living, breathing and growing area of practice encompasses four distinct approaches: the arts in health care settings, community arts in health, medical humanities and art therapy. It embraces the visual arts, performing arts, creative writing – indeed virtually every art form.

The use of the arts in health care settings does not deny anyone treatment. The money used to fund the arts cannot be used to hire additional staff. The discipline seeks to incorporate the values and perspectives of the arts and humanities into the healing environment and the very ethos of health care delivery, and at the same time to provide a value-added service for patients, visitors and staff.

Community arts in health projects both directly and indirectly impact upon the lives of local citizens and the communities they form. The arts can provide a powerful way to communicate messages that local authorities and health authorities have traditionally sought to share through leaflets and brochures. Importantly, the impact of those messages is often longer-lasting when delivered in these innovative ways.

The medical humanities are changing the way patients, families and health care professionals communicate about health. Through the humanities, medical practitioners gain a clearer understanding of the patient's experience and, in turn, the patient acquires insight into the motivation and passion of the 'hand that heals'. Literature, philosophy, drama, the visual arts, as well as more contemporary art forms such as film and television, have opened pathways for dialogue and given voice to the unknown science of the human spirit.

Art therapy has now been recognised by the Department of Health as a valuable part of health care provision. Art therapists require a postgraduate degree and must be registered in order to practice. Psychological issues are addressed through the arts and through other creative activities. The fine line between the therapeutic benefits of the arts and the arts as therapy offers challenges, with art therapy and the broader field of arts in health now beginning to come together, learning from one another and pooling resources to work towards common goals and objectives.

Which again begs the question, why isn't there more of it? One answer is that while government and non-government bodies alike now recognise the value of dialogue between the arts and health sectors, there remains a fundamental lack of investment. Money will only be forthcoming once the evidence of the effectiveness of arts-based health interventions is available. Whilst many working within this field view the results of their work as self-evident, it is now clear that funders, including, crucially, service providers, do require a persuasive evidence base before they will commit any money.

On top of the solid foundation of good practice, the evidence base is now building. Literature reviews, evaluations, and research studies are being undertaken to collate the increasing number of testimonies that arts and health together heal better than either can alone. Whether anecdotal evidence, such as a nurse commenting that blood pressure levels are lower in patients in the presence of live music on an intensive care ward, or scientifically monitored studies showing a lower need for analgesics when patients are treated within a setting with an arts programme, the field is beginning to gather the data it needs.

I believe that no one, given the choice, would actively prefer to be treated in a health care setting devoid of the arts, or to live in a community with no arts in health provision. Nor, I believe, would anyone prefer to be treated by a medical practitioner unaware of humanities issues, or to be treated in a healthcare setting where the option of art therapy is simply not available. This book takes us a step closer to appreciating why, and will hopefully bring any readers previously unconvinced of the potential of arts and humanities to improve health and well-being a step closer to saying, 'I just don't understand why there isn't more of it.'

LARA DOSE
Director, National Network of the Arts in Health
October 2003

1

The healing environment: without and within

DEBORAH KIRKLIN

This book argues the importance of the arts in the creation of physical and conceptual space supportive of healing and health. In this opening chapter Dr Deborah Kirklin, a general practitioner and senior lecturer in medical humanities, introduces a framework for thinking about the interplay between the many determinants of health and well-being.

Advances in modern medicine have done much to alleviate human suffering. Nevertheless, the fundamental importance of the wider context or environment within which patients experience illness, and the physical embodiment of that experience, can all too easily be overlooked or sidelined in an increasingly scientific approach to health care. In this chapter I will discuss a number of different facets of this environment: *physical*, *social*, *psychological*, and *person-to-person*. I will offer examples, like those which appear throughout this book, of how the arts can beneficially affect each of these, interrelated, environments.

Physical, social, psychological and person-to-person environments

Although climate and the natural world affect health, the physical environment with which I am here concerned is the man-made one. Nor do I intend to consider the impact of man-made environmental damage on health, although this is clearly very important, and a subject of legitimate concern for practitioners and for scholars of medical humanities.[1]

In this chapter I am, instead, interested in the physical environment created by human actions, thoughts or minds, that is otherwise known as human culture. This includes the built environment, both in the community and in health care settings, and the arts themselves. The importance of these settings, and the cultural resources they contain, is discussed elsewhere in this volume.*

The social environment which humans inhabit is shaped by family, by friends, by work, and by societal expectations and taboos. In *The illness narratives*, psychiatrist and anthropologist Arthur Kleinman describes how this social environment informs the way we react to and interpret illness. 'Local cultural orientations (the patterned ways we have learned to think about and act in our life worlds) organise our conventional common sense about how to understand and treat illness; thus we can say of illness that it is always culturally shaped'.[2] In other words, our social environment shapes our psychological environment in a way that, in turn, shapes our response to illness.

That illness is always culturally shaped is echoed in Arthur Frank's analysis of how illness is currently experienced in Western culture. In *The wounded storyteller*, Frank explains that 'the *modern* experience of illness begins when popular experience is overtaken by technical experience, including complex organisations of treatment'.[3] He goes on to explain that instead of going to bed and dying, cared for by friends and family, people now go to paid professionals 'who reinterpret their pains as symptoms, using a specialised language that is unfamiliar and overwhelming'. 'Illness becomes a *circulation of stories* professional and lay, but not all stories are equal.' In the modern period the story or narrative that the medical professional tells about the illness trumps all others. Frank goes on to say that 'The *postmodern* experience of illness begins when ill people recognise that more is involved in their experience than medical stories tell'.†

---

*See Chapters 2, 4, 5 and 6 by John Wells-Thorpe, Ghislaine Kenyon, Rosalia Staricoff and Susan Loppert, and Jane Duncan.

†Practitioners do not, of course, exist in isolation from the world and social change: Roger Higgs argues in this book that changes in the doctor-patient relationship are being shaped as much by changes in the expectations of doctors as by those of patients.

The internal, psychological environment through which our view of life is refracted is the starting point for all human experience, the place where self-conscious human beings try to make sense of their bodily experiences. Arthur Kleinman defines illness as 'the lived experience of monitoring bodily processes such as respiratory wheezes, abdominal cramps...' He goes on to define illness problems as 'the principal difficulties that symptoms and disability create in our lives': 'illness complaints are what patients and their families bring to their practitioners' and 'disease is what the practitioner creates in the recasting of illness in terms of theories of disorder'.

The nature of the illness the practitioner is offered for reshaping depends not only on the cultural determinants mentioned above, but also on the way in which human culture casts illness as a problem, or not. This analysis accords with the social model of disability, which acknowledges that societal attitudes, priorities and organisation are strong determinants of what Kleinman calls 'illness problems'.[2] According to the social model of disability, a person who is unable to see a movie because there isn't space for a wheelchair in the cinema is disabled not by their inability to walk (the medical explanation of disability) but by the lack of wheelchair access to the cinema.

People who are ill face the challenge of reconciling the medical and social worlds they find themselves inhabiting even during severe illness and hospitalisation. Frank identifies as a weakness in the practice of modern medicine the failure to include, as a core task, 'helping people to think differently about their post-illness worlds and construct new relationships to those worlds'.[3] This work should begin early on in an illness, not as an afterthought. The term 'post-illness' merits further consideration if we are to fully understand Frank's point. From a medical perspective, a patient is 'post-illness', or no longer ill, once a disease is cured. In contrast, Frank's use of the term post-illness does not turn on whether the person remains ill or not. Frank is referring to any time in a person's life that is lived after they first become ill, in contrast to their life before they became ill.

This use of the term acknowledges the fact that patients continue to live with the consequences of their illness – whether physical, social, psychological, economic or occupational – even after medical cure or remission has been achieved. The arts offer a way of helping people to think differently about their post-illness worlds and construct new relationships to those worlds, whether it be through arts therapies like the poetry described by John Fox in Chapter 11, or through community arts programmes like the Mind Arts Project in Stockport (MAPS), the mental health arts programme described by Michael Anderson in Chapter 7. In this way people can find their own ways of living the life they have to the full.

Andrew Mawson, who has played an active role in using the arts to regenerate a community, speaks of another important environment, 'a person-to-person environment' where people work creatively together.[4] The challenge for patients, families, doctors and other health care professionals is to develop person-to-person environments within health care that are based on a shared understanding of what matters.

Can the arts help to create a healthy environment?

In 1999 and 2001 the Nuffield Trust,[5] under the auspices of their chairman John Wyn Owen, organised invited conferences to bring together representatives of all those working, across the UK, with the arts and humanities in relation to health. These meetings included representatives from arts therapy, arts in health, community arts and medical education. The results of these important meetings, including a statement of future aims for the arts in health, *The Windsor Declaration*, can be found in publications by the Trust.[4,6] The meetings tried to map out the many and varied ways in which the arts and humanities can influence health and well-being, and succeeded in attracting the interest and attention of the wider medical establishment, the lay public and policy-makers. Importantly, practical ways in which the arts could improve health were sought, and recommendations for future work to develop the potential of the field were offered. The arts in health, community arts, art therapies, and medical humanities were identified as areas of particular interest.

The report of the first conference anticipated wide-ranging health gains if the arts and humanities were raised to a pivotal role in health care.[6] The gains included:

▷ more compassionate, intuitive doctors and other health professionals;

▷ patient empowerment through creative expression;

> ▷ reduced dependence on psychotropic medication such as tranquillisers and anti-depressants;

> ▷ growing confidence and self-reliance of individuals and communities; and,

> ▷ the provision of an approach and support to help combat social exclusion.

The nature and scope of the anticipated health gains make it clear that health is not determined only by the medical care someone receives when sick, but by the life that person lives beyond, and in parallel with, their interactions with doctors and the health care system in the post-illness world that Frank describes.

Caring for the person: the without and the within

In the 1980s, the Government introduced the policy of care in the community.[7] Health authorities, responding to the obligation to move long-term patient care from inpatient settings to the community whenever possible, closed many long-term health care institutions. Many long-term, often institutionalised, in-patients found themselves back in the community. The sad, black joke amongst medics at the time was that the idea was sound in principle, but that unfortunately there no longer was a community, and certainly not a caring one.

Despite on-going concerns about how much capacity for care exists in the community, it is a daily reality for health care providers that socialised medicine appears inadequate to the task of replacing the care that a vibrant community can offer. Medical and social services are often overwhelmed by seemingly endless demands – the situation is, sadly, highlighted when system failures lead to tragedy.* So knowing about and caring about what happens out in the community should be highly important to health care providers, not only those working in the community but also those in secondary and tertiary institutions.

The development of arts in community settings ('community arts') aims to empower individuals and communities through

---

*Victoria Climbié, for example, was an eight-year-old girl who died of abuse despite several different health and social services being aware of her case. For information about this tragic episode see **www.victoria-climbie-inquiry.org.uk**

creative expression, to encourage confidence and self-reliance in individuals and communities, and thereby to provide an important means of combating social exclusion. One community arts approach involves accessing existing resources. An interesting example of this is the work of the National Gallery's Education Department, described in Chapter 4 by Ghislaine Kenyon. Another approach involves projects such as MAPS, a community arts project designed specifically with the needs of a group of individuals in mind; in the case of MAPS those with mental health problems (Chapter 7). Alternatively, community arts may involve community regeneration programmes which use the arts as a way of building confidence, self-reliance and social cohesion.

The Bromley by Bow project provides a flourishing example of just that. Andrew Mawson, the project's founder, says, 'At the Bromley by Bow Centre in the East End of London, over the last 15 years, we've tried to pioneer healthy living centres and have connected GPs with arts, with parks, and with housing... It is all based on an organic model of backing people before structures... We find centres of energised people and back them with real money so that they can expand and multiply and form relationships with each other. We trust in them and they just get on with it.'[4]

Andrew Mawson is acutely aware of the importance of the environment in which people are asked to find creative solutions to problems: 'Instinct tells me that you can't put new things into old environments... for example, anyone wanting to start a healthy living centre is put directly in touch with someone who has actually built one, so you start to create a person-to-person environment where decisions can be made today and acted on tomorrow. We [the Community Action Network, a national charity of which Andrew is director] now [have] 2,000 people all trying to build this new environment.'[8]

The importance of the built environment in human flourishing has also long been recognised by architects and the public. Indeed, purpose built health care settings have a considerable history. This is acknowledged in Chapters 2 and 3 by John Wells Thorpe and Ruth Richardson. As John reports, the impact of the built environment on the experiences of hospital inpatients can be objectively measured, and it is likely that the impact is seldom neutral.

The arts in health is now a flourishing and vibrant field which brings art, including visual art, performance and live music, into health care settings. The appeal is to the general human interest in, and need for, the arts and all they have to offer. This does not abate just because people are temporarily forced by ill health to leave their communities. Here therapy, whilst often welcome, could be argued to be an incidental rather than primary objective.

Yet these seemingly incidental effects are now the subject of increasing interest and research. Rosalia Staricoff and Susan Loppert report on studies which show that the arts in health can have a positive impact on clinical outcomes in a variety of clinical settings (Chapter 5). The anxiety and depression levels of in-patients can be reduced, and interestingly, the existence of a lively arts programme within a hospital seems to have a positive impact on staff retention and recruitment. Research undertaken by Jane Duncan shows that the different colours she used to create public art in a hydrotherapy pool evoked very specific emotional responses in users. Her work, described in Chapter 6, underlines the need for care in the choice of colours used in these settings.

The therapeutic use of the creative arts with patients, carers and professionals (known as art therapy) has a long and respected tradition. The use of poetry therapy, a fine example of this work, is described by John Fox in Chapter 11 and in his book *Poetic medicine*.[9]

Entering each other's worlds: a medical humanities approach*

The vast majority of doctors, would-be doctors, and other health care professionals, are, I believe, caring individuals trying to do a good job for the people entrusted to their care. But sometimes, as we all know, even caring and competent individuals can end up doing a less than ideal job, and it is important to ask why. Perhaps sometimes it's because the doctor or nurse has simply failed to appreciate what it is that the patient needs, feels and wants; what their priorities are.

---

*The scope of medical humanities is far and wide. In the UK, this is still a rapidly evolving area and so no one view can define it. My own definition of medical humanities is of an inter-disciplinary, and increasingly international, endeavour that draws on the creative and intellectual strengths of diverse disciplines, including literature, art, creative writing, drama, film, music, philosophy, ethical decision-making, anthropology and history, in pursuit of medical educational goals.

Or perhaps it's because they appreciate what the patient needs, feels and wants all too well, and they simply don't know how to deal with the combined burden of the patient's pain and their own.[10,11]

Several contributors to this volume offer examples of ways in which literature can help practitioners gain a better understanding of the experience of illness (either as patient or carer), and of the unique world view that shapes decisions people make with regard to lifestyle and health. Claire Elliott describes how contemporary fiction can be used to assist health care professionals in understanding health decisions that at first glance seem to make no sense. Michele Petrone offers an insight into how serious illness, and the loneliness and powerlessness of institutionalised health care, created its own nightmare for him: a real nightmare which allowed him to gain a fresh perspective on his own experience and which, shared, may help others in a similar predicament (Chapter 9). Finally Michael Rowe, a father and a sociologist, shares with us the pain and understanding that came from caring for his dying child (Chapter 10). His essay serves as a reminder to all practitioners that they too will one day be recipients rather than providers of care. In this sense he provides us all with a serious and personal incentive to listen well.

When it comes to an experience as intensely personal as illness, and decisions about health behaviour, even the most empathetic doctor will never be able to understand fully what the patient is going through. Nevertheless the arts and medicine can allow a vicarious understanding through empathy.[12] Robert Cole has argued that stories can exercise and sensitise the moral imagination of those who engage with them.[13] Lois Nixon, describing the use of literature in the education of medical students, has observed that 'the approach is postmodernist; we walk around the subject listening to several voices, perspectives, interpretations. The non-medical materials move students away from textbook descriptions and analysis, forcing them to discover connections, to re-vision ways of knowing what we know'.[14]

Conclusion

This book sets out to give substance to the claim that the arts and humanities can help foster a physical, social, psychological, and person-to-person environment which is supportive of health and well-being, or human flourishing. For patients and health care practitioners, understanding the nature of the environment that any individual occupies is a necessary prelude to devising and agreeing appropriate health strategies. The arts offer a means to a shared understanding between patients and practitioners of what matters, and the creation of a person-to-person environment supportive of both parties. The arts can help re-shape the physical environment so that it enables people to live their lives to the full. The arts can help rebuild a community based on trust and confidence, and the arts can foster creative exploration of and reflection on the inner worlds that all of us inhabit.

References

1 Special Issue: Environment and Health. *Literature and Medicine* 1996;**15**(1):1–146.

2 Kleinman A. *The illness narratives*. New York, NY: Basic Books, 1988.

3 Frank A. *The wounded storyteller*. Chicago, MI: University of Chicago Press, 1997.

4 Philipp R. *Arts, health, and well being*. London: Nuffield Trust, 2002.

5 **www.nuffieldtrust.org.uk**

6 Philipp R, Baum M, Mawson A, Calman K. *Humanities in medicine: beyond the millennium*. London: Nuffield Trust, 1999.

7 National Health Service and Community Care Act, 1990 (c. 19).

8 **www.can-online.org.uk**

9 Fox J. *Poetic medicine*. New York: Putnam, 1997.

10 Clark L. A piece of my mind. Joshua knew. *JAMA* 1993;**270**(24):2902.

11 Schultz S. A father's eyes. *JAMA* 1995;**271**(15):1146.

12 Kirklin D, Meakin R, Singh S, Lloyd M. 'Living with and dying from cancer': a humanities special study module. *J Med Ethics: Medical Humanities* 2000;**26**:51–54.

13 Cole R. *The call of stories: teaching and the moral imagination*. Boston MA: Houghton Mifflin, 1989.

14 Nixon LL, 'Medical humanities: pyramids and rhomboids in the rationalist world of medicine.' In Lindemann Nelson H (ed). *Stories and their limits*. New York: Routledge, 1997.

2

Healing by design: feeling better?

JOHN WELLS-THORPE

John Wells-Thorpe, architect and health service chairman, demonstrates that the built environment of health care can affect the length of inpatient stays and patients' evaluations of staff and quality of care received. His research highlights the importance of user consultation before new building or renovation, and argues that patients value control of their environment as much as aesthetics.

Introduction

This chapter describes a three-year research project aimed at assessing the impact of a planned change in health care setting for two groups of hospital inpatients. The work involved clinical teams, managers, architects and external researchers drawn from two NHS trusts – one acute (orthopaedic) and the other community (mental health) – and Sheffield University School of Architecture. As a practising architect appointed to chair one of the first NHS trusts, I had decided that more work should be undertaken to see whether measurable therapeutic benefit could be derived from better design. I therefore assembled the team and obtained research funding for the project.

Background

Anecdotal evidence concerning the probable effect of a patient's surroundings abounds. Some of the first allusions occur in fifteenth century Italy, where there was felt to be a strong correlation between illness and spirituality, and where physicians were perceived as instruments of God. Epidemics of plague and syphilis afflicted large sections of the community, and religious communities, acting as servants of Christ, provided early hospices or hospitals.

'Buildings are important more as a setting for human life than as works of art.'

Sir Peter Shepheard

These caring communities were at pains to provide the best available patient care. The hospitals they built had high ceilings to allow natural ventilation to exhaust the 'corrupt and disease-carrying air', as it was once described. Such buildings incidentally provided large wall areas ideal for frescoes, of which the most famous were in Santa Maria della Scala in Siena in the fifteenth century. Leading artists and sculptors from the region were employed. The church-like appearance of the buildings was further enhanced by a conspicuous altar, positioned so that patients could see the Mass during times of distress.[1]

Much later, on her return from Constantinople in 1859, Florence Nightingale argued for the therapeutic potential of physical environments, expressing forceful opinions on the form, colour, lighting and views of hospital wards. She wrote:

> I have seen the most acute suffering produced from a patient not being able to see out of a window. I shall never forget the rapture of fever patients over a bunch of bright-coloured flowers. People say the effect is only on the mind. It is no such thing. The effect is on the body too. Little as we know about the way in which we are affected by form, by colour, and light, we do know this, and that they have an actual physical effect.[2]

Although they are not usually incorporated into modern hospital design, many of Nightingale's ideas remain relevant today, particularly those relating to the importance of outside views and how every patient should be able to watch sunlight moving around a ward through a day.

In more recent times philosophers, writers and poets have reminded us of the powerful influences which can be exerted on individuals by their physical environment. The twentieth century philosopher Ludwig Wittgenstein remarked: 'Remember the impression one gets from good architecture, that it expresses a *thought*.'[3]

Contemporary health care settings can sometimes appear impersonal, conveying a sense of a controlling regime and making the patient feel alienated. Unfortunately, as a sociologist colleague pointed out, the hospital bed can be perceived by patients not as a safe haven, but rather as a medium of containment which renders the patient a passive object of clinicians' activity.

In the last twenty years there has been an increase in the still-limited amount of research being undertaken internationally in this field. Research at the Chelsea and Westminster Hospital, described elsewhere in this volume, seeks to evaluate the deliberate integration of the arts in a hospital environment, and raises fundamental questions about whether the visual arts and performance can play a meaningful role in health care.* At the Norwegian University of Science and Technology in Trondheim, Professor Arnulf Kolstad is assessing patients' visual perception of architecture in psychiatric wards. He claims that architecture and the built environment trigger certain states of awareness and can evoke a variety of personal associations. Physical appearance, geometrical forms, colours, fixtures and furniture therefore affect the atmosphere of the ward, with these physical properties of the built environment symbolising the values and treatment ideologies.[4]

Another relatively unexplored, but potentially important, area of research and therapy involves the use of virtual reality. At the University of Washington Medical School, Seattle, a symptom-control procedure has been tried in an acute burns unit. Patients spent half an hour in a virtual reality studio, looking at a scene of dusk in Antarctica, as shadows lengthen across the frozen landscape, and the wind induces a blizzard. Patients experiencing acute discomfort from their burns and skin grafts derive genuine relief from their symptoms as a result of this treatment.

Like other intriguing experiments in this field, this finding raises the additional question of the extent to which illusion can be used as a therapeutic tool. Similarly, we need to know a lot more about the role and value of *distraction* in health care design, mindful of TS Eliot's reflection that 'humankind cannot bear too much reality'.[5]

Healing by design: the nature of the problem

In the UK, £2–3 billion is spent annually on the built estate in the NHS. Despite many attempts in the recent past to improve hospital design, there is currently a growing recognition that planning efficiency, cost effectiveness, service flexibility and other criteria

---

*See Chapter 5, 'Integrating the arts into health care: can we affect clinical outcomes?' by Rosalia Staricoff and Susan Loppert.

alone do not adequately meet today's needs for patient-centred care. Quantitative issues appeal to the scientifically trained mind, whilst *qualitative* issues – which are not so easily susceptible to measurement or costing – are sometimes considered inappropriate considerations in hospital design. Such factors are often regarded as subjective, and can easily be dismissed as supported only by anecdotal evidence and therefore imprecise and peripheral.

A strong argument can, however, be made that the qualitative aspects of the built environment are far from peripheral; that they are central to patients' experiences. Inpatients spend a great deal of time with little to do. Patients in hospital may get the personal attention of a doctor for only a few minutes in a day, with only slightly longer periods of care from nurses and therapists. For the rest of the time, however, they lie in bed, sit, get wheeled about or walk around in their environment. I would argue that this relatively inactive and static environment makes them potentially far more sensitive to the environment than those who aren't hospitalised and are free to change their environment by moving around. It seems reasonable, therefore, to ask in what ways the built environment may affect patients' sense of well-being, and whether it can influence their recovery, either for good or for bad.

It is also important to remember that the internal arrangements of health care settings should be designed primarily for patient-centred, rather than staff-centred, reasons. Unfortunately, many health care buildings encode social and hierarchical structures within their design. All too frequently the hospital setting reinforces the power and dominion of health professionals, and patients can be left feeling undervalued or that, as I heard of one protesting, 'a patient is a person and not a barcode'.

The research remit

In 1999, I was invited to form a research team to examine the effect of the built environment on the therapeutic process. An important outcome was to be the formulation of a new set of guidelines which could be of value to others designing health care settings throughout the NHS. The research project was entitled 'The architectural healthcare environment and its effects on patient health outcomes'. It was funded by a three-year grant from the UK Government.

Two NHS trusts that were planning to move existing cohorts of patients from old accommodation into new were identified. One, at Poole, Dorset, involved acute sector inpatients (orthopaedic) and the other, at Brighton, Sussex, involved non-acute sector inpatients (mental health). In both cases, whilst the health care *setting* changed, the clinical and managerial regime and staff remained the same, as did the treatment and medication. Whilst a considerable number of patients moved from old accommodation to new at both Poole and Brighton, the remainder of those being studied had either only been in the old accommodation or were fresh admissions to the new. In a small number of cases in Brighton, there were some re-admissions after a period of time spent in the community; these patients therefore experienced both old and new settings, but with an interval of time in between.

Patients' views on a number of aspects of the built environment were elicited before and after the moves. We were particularly interested in patient views on the quality of the built environment including: overall general appearance, satisfaction with specific spaces (both personal and communal), lighting, temperature, air quality, noise, and perceived levels of individual control over the physical environment. We were also interested to know whether patients felt the environment affected their sense of well-being in any way, and whether their assessment of the quality of the care they received, and the staff providing it, was affected. Every effort was made to ensure that patients felt free to express their views on all these matters. Other more easily quantifiable health outcomes were also monitored, including length of inpatient stay, anxiety levels, patient satisfaction with care received, and use of pain medication. The fieldwork was observed by the University of Sheffield School of Architecture, under the direction of Professor Bryan Lawson.[6] Work is currently going on to evaluate the cost implications of the design considerations of this study.

The two settings for the study

Poole

The Poole project (the orthopaedic part of the study) involved the refurbishment of existing 1960s acute general wards. In the original ward there were six four-bed bays and six one-bed bays, with lavatories at each end of the ward. In the refurbished unit there are 16 single bedrooms and three four-bed bays. The new bedrooms have a clean, simple interior (using natural timber), and en-suite bathrooms.

Brighton

The Brighton project (the mental health part of the study) involved the replacement of two 15-bed communal wards in Brighton General Hospital in Victorian brick buildings with typically high ceilings, by a new purpose-built mental health unit, Mill View Hospital, accommodating a 32-bed unit with single rooms, and en-suite facilities.

The design process

We first held focus groups with a series of people involved in the commissioning, management, design and daily use of these kinds of buildings, because we needed to know what the clients' expectations were, the design teams' intentions, and what was thought to be important among experienced users of such buildings.

From work with these focus groups, we were able to formulate the questionnaires which would be offered to patients at the end of their stay. The questionnaires were intended to elicit their reactions to the building and the treatment they had received, and allow assessments by the staff caring for them. It was decided that, in the case of the mentally ill patients, we would arrange the questionnaires through their carers. Patients in general were happy to take part in the study, and were encouragingly forthcoming and articulate about their views concerning their environment.

The architectural remit

Poole

The architects, Llewellyn Davies, were asked to design an efficient and life-enhancing environment for patients and staff alike, and to break away from the geometric rigours of functional 1960s buildings. They did this by punctuating the internal spaces with design features, and introducing curved walls in suitable locations to relieve the monotomy of the basic structure.

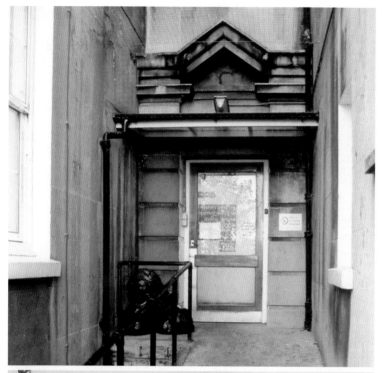

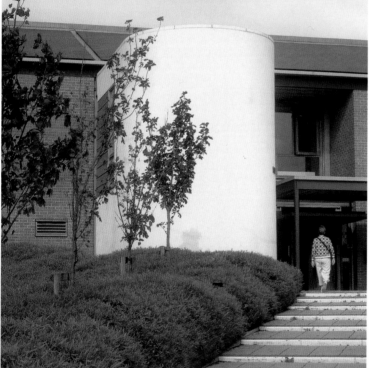

Top: The entrance to the old mental health care unit at Brighton General Hospital.

Bottom: The entrance to the new mental health care unit at Mill View Hospital, Brighton.

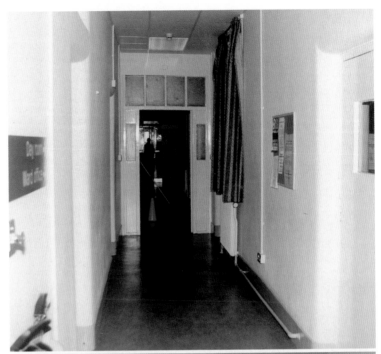

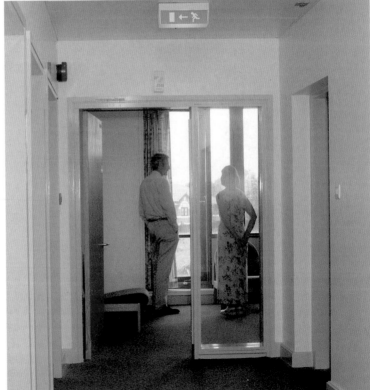

Top: A corridor ending in darkness and gloom in former accommodation at Brighton General Hospital.

Bottom: A corridor ending in light and a view at the new Mill View Hospital, Brighton.

Brighton

The appointed architects, Powell and Moya, having been selected by competition, were asked to consider the most effective ways of using colour, natural light, texture, spatial continuity and land-scaping to provide a humane and personalised environment for patients. They were shown the old, nineteenth century buildings which were in use. This was a very demanding remit because of the often conflicting need for security on the one hand and rapid escape from fire on the other.

The illustrations which accompany this chapter demonstrate the dramatic contrast between the old and new accommodation at Brighton.

Research findings

Patients in the newer buildings expressed greater satisfaction with the appearance, layout and overall design of their wards.[6] At Poole Hospital, 72% of the patients in the new unit gave the highest rating they could for overall appearance, compared with only 37% of the patients in the old unit. At Brighton both these figures were lower, with 41% giving the highest rating for the new unit compared with only 20% for the old. Despite the generally lower satisfaction figures in the case of mental health patients, there was still a significant increase in satisfaction ratings.

Specific spaces in the newer buildings were also more highly praised. The most significant differences were in the patients' assessment of their own 'private area', whether in a multiple bed bay or a single room.[6]

Patients were asked detailed questions about specific aspects of their physical environment, including lighting, temperature, air quality and noise. In both settings the new buildings tended to be more highly-rated than the old, although the differences were less marked than those for overall design and spatial organisation. Next, we asked what levels of control patients had over aspects of their environment, such as being able to turn off lights, open windows and alter heating, and replies indicated that patients in both settings were clearly unhappy with this aspect, reporting low levels of control over their environment in both the old and new buildings. We concluded that inadequate consideration was given to these aspects at the design briefing stage.

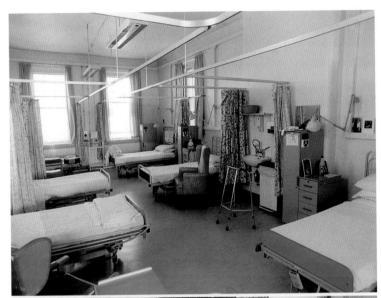

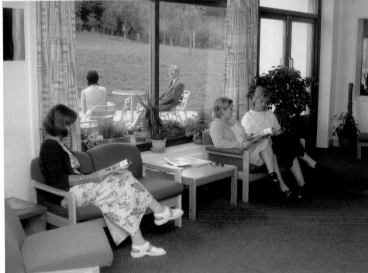

Top: Spatial containment and clutter at former mental health care unit, Brighton General Hospital.

Bottom: Spatial continuity and order at the new mental health care unit, Mill View Hospital, Brighton.

Patients in the old and new buildings at both locations were asked whether they thought the environment had helped them feel better. In both the Poole and Brighton settings, the move resulted in a significant improvement in patients' assessments of their new surroundings. We also asked patients to gauge the overall quality of their treatment, and to 'rate' the staff who had cared for them. In both cases we found an improvement in these ratings in the newer buildings, although these differences were not always statistically significant.[6] Remarkably, in the newer environments patients thought they had received better treatment, and that their doctors, nurses and therapists were more helpful and attentive. This revealing finding merits further study.

On direct questioning concerning positive and negative features of the environment, two major groups or clusters of factors emerged as important to patients. The first and most obvious concern has to do with direct relationships between people and their environment, including factors such as the colours of surfaces or the temperature of rooms. The second group of factors concerns the manner in which the environment mediates relationships between people, and includes matters of privacy, whether people are able to establish community or maintain 'personal space'.

It is often assumed that the value of 'good design' lies largely in the first category, perceived in aesthetic or functional terms. Our results did not support this assumption. The most commonly raised issue amongst all four of our patient samples was that of privacy, which is not to say that all our respondents were asking to be entirely private. Nevertheless, the manner in which the environment enabled or inhibited privacy or sociability seemed to be of the greatest importance to our patients. Such social factors – perhaps reflecting a natural desire to retain a modicum of autonomy despite hospitalisation – are easily overlooked in environments not consciously designed to be patient-centred.

Next in order of importance to patients was the view, or outlook, available to them. The most common complaint made during the course of the study was the lack of any significant view. Nurses and others working in the hospitals also mentioned this problem, both for themselves and for their patients. There was no evidence that, in general, patients wanted classically beautiful views. The desire, rather, was for views of everyday life in which normal events occurred, such as children leaving school or the changing colour of the sea, and which would encourage conversation between patients about unfolding events outside.

Health outcomes

Our study looked at a number of health outcomes in each location. In both Poole and Brighton, inpatients' discharge time was significantly improved from the new wards compared to the old ones. In the general medical wards at Poole, patients who did not undergo operations were discharged on average one and a half days earlier from the new wards. This represents a reduction of about 21% in the average length of stay. There was also a dramatic reduction in the amount of analgesic medication taken by the patients on the newer wards.[6]

In the new mental health care setting at Brighton, a reduction of 14% was recorded in the length of inpatient stay. Patients were judged by staff to be significantly less aggressive, making fewer verbal outbursts and showing fewer instances of threatening behaviour, and the number of instances of patients injuring themselves was reduced by two-thirds. Most dramatically, the amount of time patients needed to spend in secluded accommodation was reduced by 70%. Overall, the result was a calmer and less hostile environment, with patients making better progress and being discharged earlier.

Conclusion

The study yielded two interesting conclusions, which have important implications for others working in this field.

First, being able to control the environment and decide what levels of privacy and community are wanted by individuals is extremely important to patients in hospital. Meeting these needs by means of hospital design leads not only to higher levels of general satisfaction, but also to a significant improvement in satisfaction with the medical treatment received. Such qualitative data provides compelling evidence that matters of privacy versus community, and personal control over the environment, are of fundamental importance to patients; indeed of greater significance to them than the general appearance or aesthetics of those surroundings.

Secondly, this study shows that improving the built environment can reduce the length of inpatient stay times, reduce the need for analgesia, and improve patients' perceptions both of the quality of care they have received and the quality of the staff caring for them.

The study shows that improving the nature of the built environment could have beneficial cost implications, and improve patients' experiences of hospital. It is hoped that this work, which combined qualitative and quantitative approaches, will provide inspiration and encouragement to architects, clinicians, managers and patients to work together to ensure the environments they build promote health and well-being.

References

1   Marsh H. Paper at a conference on 'Building a better patient environment'. The Prince's Foundation, November 2001.

2   Nightingale F. *Notes on nursing: what it is and what it is not*. New York: Dover Publications, 1969.

3   Wittgenstein L. *Culture and value*. Oxford: Blackwell Publishers, 1998.

4   Kolstad A, Bjornsen P. First impressions of atmosphere in psychiatric acute wards – associations from visual perception of architecture. A paper presented at the 'Human centred design for health care buildings', first international conference, August 1997, Trondheim, Norway.

5   Eliot TS. *Four quartets*. London: Faber, 1936.

6   Lawson B, Wells-Thorpe J. *The architectural healthcare environment and its effects on patient health outcomes*. Sheffield: NHS Estates/Stationery Office, 2003.

3

Building healing environments: an historical perspective

RUTH RICHARDSON

Historian Ruth Richardson reminds us of the rich history of the physical environment and ethos of health service institutions. Many present-day hospitals are mediaeval in origin, others were 'voluntary' or charitable foundations, teaching hospitals, or Victorian Poor Law infirmaries. Future health care environments should take the good and reject the bad from the learning curve of the past.

My first visit to the new Chelsea and Westminster Hospital in London's Fulham Road was a revelation. It was magnificent. It felt so completely different to the dark, forbidding, dingy and gaunt building which had been there before. This was light, bright, vibrant, welcoming – and it was quite unlike my own mental image of 'hospital'.

The height and brilliance of the hospital's inner atrium felt to me like a modern incarnation of a great mediaeval cathedral (lofty gothic columns, deceptively delicate fan vaulting, upper clerestories of light) *amalgamated* with a handsome cloister – a refuge of greenery and tranquil open space in the midst of the booming of bells, the collective hum of services, and the whisperings of prayers.

Those great mediaeval edifices were circled with side chapels, dedicated to specific saints, while the hospital has its departments dedicated to particular organs, systems or treatments of the human body. And while in a cathedral the seats of the confessionals awaited priests and penitents, here the various consulting rooms serve patients and professionals in a building beneficently dedicated to the comfort of visitors in this world rather than the next.

My pleasure in its architectural splendour was influenced in part by the notion of 'hospital' with which I had grown up. The word conjured up a place which more closely resembled the old building which had been demolished to make way for the construction of this new one.

The Knacker's Yard

I'd known the old St Stephen's Hospital, Fulham Road, only by its massive, dark, daunting exterior. It was one of those buildings which embodied all that was really grim about the Victorian era, one of those buildings you didn't enter unless you had to. Its dismal facade infected the atmosphere of the street outside for quite a distance, even in the 1960s, with a sombre Marley's Ghost sort of an atmosphere. The temperature seemed to drop as you walked through its shadow, as did one's spirits. Its close resemblance to other hospitals, built in what were to their Victorian builders the hinterlands of London, meant I had a feeling that I knew its interior atmosphere inside out.

My family goes back six generations in north Kensington, a part of London not unlike the Fulham Road. Both districts are now regarded as central, and very fashionable – so much so that the children of long-standing inhabitants cannot afford to remain. But until comparatively recently, both neighbourhoods had large populations of indigenous working class poor, and the hospitals which served them were ex-Poor Law institutions.

The one nearest us was (and actually still is) known to its clientele as the 'Knacker's Yard'. The story was that if you went in there, you never came out alive. As a child I was told by other children in my school playground that when the hospital chimney was smoking, they were disposing of patients.

Before the Appointed Day in 1948 when the 'Knacker's Yard' was adopted by the National Health Service, it wasn't a hospital but a workhouse infirmary. Most people nowadays wouldn't know that these two types of institution were historically quite distinct, or that until the twentieth century they served different patients.

Voluntary hospitals

Generally speaking, 'hospitals' were 'voluntary' or teaching hospitals, supported by charitable funds and donations, with boards of governors and illustrious trustees. Medical posts were much sought after, because staff gained great prestige by association with these hospitals, which in turn greatly enhanced their income from private patients. If the hospital was a teaching institution doctors also received students' fees.

Hospitals tended to be architecturally memorable insofar as they had noble buildings with pleasing details (often classical in derivation) such as columns, pilasters, pediments and porticoes. They were invariably faced with stone or terracotta, and had decorative ironwork, occasional stone-carved detailing, or, less frequently, statuary. They were usually situated in places conveniently near to main roads and city centres.

They admitted injured and acutely ill patients through casualty. Other 'interesting' cases for a long time had to prove that they were also 'respectable' and 'deserving' by obtaining letters from charitable subscribers.

Hospitals had neither the space nor facilities for patients suffering from chronic or terminal illnesses. Their interest was in a high turnover of patients, so as to provide impressive annual statistics of 'cases successfully treated', and thereby to sustain the interest of subscribers and attract further charitable donations. Florence Nightingale knew that Victorian hospital managers massaged these statistics: 'We have known incurable cases discharged from one hospital, to which the deaths should been accounted, and received into another hospital, to die there in a day or two'.[1] The Poor Law offered hospitality of a sort to the hopeless poor. 'Those who are turned out of the London hospitals, go to the workhouses to die,' said another Victorian observer.[2]

Workhouse infirmaries

The patients in workhouse infirmaries were there not only because they were sick, but because they were poor. Had they been wealthy they would have been cared for at home; the wealthy never entered a hospital or an infirmary for treatment. Taken together, chronic illness, mental illness, infirmity, dementia, old age and terminal illness were the most frequent causes of poverty and destitution in the nineteenth century. The Poor Law infirmary was for the destitute, the claimant, the pauper: the *un*deserving.

The Victorian workhouse had been the creation of the New Poor

Law, enacted in 1834 to curtail public spending on poverty. Work-houses were erected by unions of parishes, funded by local taxation. They were built on cheap land, on sites which were often on the periphery of communities: inconvenience to paupers being of no concern. Workhouses were closed institutions, managed locally by 'guardians of the poor' and overseen centrally by the Poor Law Board, itself answerable to the Home Secretary. By the mid-nineteenth century, the workhouse system had become the largest civil organisation in the country, comprising some 700 institutions.

To deter applicants, the regime governing most of the work-houses was deliberately harsh, as typified in Dickens' *Oliver Twist*. Where local ratepayers appreciated the effects upon the working population of epidemics and trade cycles attitudes could be more benign, but workhouses and their masters were generally feared and reviled.

Poor Law architecture was never lavish. Ornamentation was kept to a minimum, or ruled out altogether by local ratepayers. In London, most Poor Law buildings were stock brick, flat fronted, with plain fenestration, and often grim: 'functional rather than aesthetic'.[3]

To receive any assistance in time of need, poor people were required to live inside the workhouse, which entailed a loss of citizenship, the sale of personal belongings, the break-up of homes and separation of families. Known as 'Bastiles' by the poor (and by a host of other euphemisms), workhouses effectively imprisoned the sick, unemployed, disabled, insane and the old alongside the few fit people they were intended to deter.

It was well known that conditions in the mid-Victorian work-house were predisposed to disease, and were *far* worse than those in prisons. Hundreds of people might be accommodated in a single building. The possibility of isolating healthy inmates from sick, or of segregating patients suffering from acute, chronic, infectious or terminal illnesses, was restricted by poor accommodation and by overcrowding. Workhouses had no casualty or surgical facilities, and many lacked separate infirmary buildings, the infirmary being merely a designated ward inside the workhouse. The sheer numbers of ill and infirm people meant that even where such wards existed, sick and dying patients might be found throughout the workhouse. One Poor Law doctor described how he had to cope alone in a building in which beds, many of them shared, were packed so close together that to get out patients had to clamber to the end of their beds.[4]

A doctor gained no status from an association with a workhouse infirmary. Since expenditure in these places was low, pay was poor. Even so, there was often a competition for medical officer posts, which were awarded by competitive tender to the lowest bidder. Salaries often included a commitment to cover the costs of medicines and dressings, which meant that many patients, whatever their suffering, received no medication at all.

Food was poor and inadequate. At Andover, for example, inmates fought each other for shreds of meat adhering to the bones they had been told to crush.[5] Hygiene was deficient, and paupers were deemed to deserve no privacy: in some places, unscreened latrines were located inside workhouse wards, badly plumbed and with no toilet paper provided. Epidemics of diarrhoea and fevers were commonplace. Inevitably, mortality was high. Thomas Wakley, medical coroner, MP, and founding editor of the *Lancet*, described workhouses as 'ante-chambers of the grave'.[6]

To give proper care to these large communities of sick and dying patients, doctors of conscience suffered both overwork and financial loss. Whatever their qualifications, workhouse doctors were nominally inferior in rank to workhouse masters, which could cause friction and difficulty in the medical management of patients' cases. Doctors voicing criticism were often induced to leave. They were supported by no paid nursing staff at all. All nursing was provided by inmates at no cost.

We can glimpse what life was like in these places during Victoria's reign because, just occasionally, a scandal – like that at Andover – would erupt, and an investigation would reveal what went on behind closed doors. Rarely, a Poor Law doctor might pen a memoir,[4] a lady visitor might give evidence to a parliamentary select committee or have the temerity to publish an open letter to the President of the Poor Law Board in an attempt to shame him into changing matters.

One such courageous woman was Louisa Twining, who herself established and ran a home for epileptic and incurable women in Queen Square, which was also a training school for nurses.[7] Louisa Twining was a key figure in the Workhouse Visiting Society. She chronicled the human effects of government recruitment and low-pay policies, as she had witnessed at first hand the terrible neglect of patients in workhouses: suffering which hitherto had been ignored. She revealed the folly of saving money on nurses by employing other paupers to do the work: 'What are indeed large hospitals cannot be managed and nursed by the very class who are placed in them because of their very incapacity'. She spoke of a case in which a pauper 'nurse' terrorised and caused great misery to elderly patients under her control (the word 'care' is inappropriate here), and of other patients 'tended at their deaths by drunken nurses'. Inmate nurses were themselves usually elderly and broken-down: 'They come not to this, the lowest office which a worn-out woman can fill, till all other chances of subsistence are gone'.

Pauper nurses lived and slept in the wards, on-call 24 hours a day, all year. Their only permitted time off was to attend the workhouse chapel, and their only perk: alcohol. Their work was unremitting: 'for no sooner does one sufferer depart, than another fills the vacant bed. For work such as this which one would conceive could only be performed from the very highest of motives of duty and devotion, [the pauper nurse] receives only the House diet... and an allowance of beer and gin'.[2]

Louisa Twining argued that according noble status to the post would be the key to recruitment of good nurses, just as it was for good cleaners, perhaps a lesson we could usefully relearn today.

Hospital reform

The mid-1860s was a key period of change.

The need for hospital and nursing reform had been revealed in the Crimea during the 1850s, and Florence Nightingale's influence had been widely felt in hospital care in Britain. But workhouse infirmaries seemed exempt from the entire debate, until Ernest Hart (who would later become a celebrated editor of the *British Medical Journal*) approached the *Lancet* (by this time edited by Thomas Wakley's sons) with the idea that the journal should itself appoint a sanitary commission to investigate the state of workhouse infirmaries.

The three doctor-commissioners looked first at the workhouses of the metropolis. The *Lancet* published their reports at intervals during the 1865/6 winter,[8] laying open the magnitude of the problem, and revealing the terrible contrast between the workhouse infirmary and the charitable hospital. The *Lancet* commissioners argued that the workhouses should rightfully be understood as state hospitals, in the grip of a policy of shameful neglect.

Whereas the great charitable and teaching hospitals of the metropolis provided less than 4,000 beds, the workhouses housed about 29,000 chronically infirm and disabled, imbecile or acutely sick patients, many of them in buildings 'quite unfit for hospital purposes.'[9]

Some local and recent improvements were noted, such as the introduction of paid nurses in a few districts, but the commission cited frequent examples of neglect amounting to extreme cruelty.[9] The conclusions were damning:

> Patch up the present system as we may ... it will still continue to be a scandal and a reproach ... the State Hospitals are in workhouse wards. They are closed against observation, they pay no heed to public opinion; they pay no toll to science. They contravene the rules of hygiene; they are under the government of men [guardians and workhouse masters] profoundly ignorant of hospital rules ... The doctor and patient alike are the object of a pinching parsimony. There is neither uniformity, nor liberality, nor intelligence in the management.[8]

Publication caused a national furore. The Government swiftly announced its own investigation, which subsequently confirmed the commission's findings, and paved the way for change.

The *British Medical Journal* reported in 1870, for example, that Dr Dudfield of St Margaret's Workhouse, Kensington, was able to report a number of substantial improvements in the workhouse since the appointment of paid day and night nurses, under the charge of a paid head-nurse. These included a diminished death rate (from 18.6% to 14.3% on the average daily number of inmates), amounting to 167 fewer deaths over the previous five years than 'had the former death rate continued'. Alcohol consumption in the house had dropped, and there was a good supply of hot water, and of fuel for warming the building:

> Among the minor but by no means insignificant reforms, is mentioned the ornamentation of the sick and infirm wards

by coloured limewash and pictures, instead of the dreary waste of bare white which must formerly have added to the depression of the patients.[10]

The fact that such things were mentioned as 'improvements' reveals what the place was like before: no proper nursing, high death rate, cold, dismal. The adoption of such improvements was neither general nor national, but piecemeal and local, down to the initiative of local enthusiasts. This meant it was lacking or only slowly accepted in many places. The Victorian poet WE Henley described his induction as an infirmary patient thus:

> my confidence all gone,
> The grey-haired soldier-porter waves me on,
> And on I crawl, and still my spirits fail:
> A tragic meanness seems so to environ
> These corridors and stairs of stone and iron,
> Cold, naked, clean – half-workhouse and half-jail.[11]

At the time Henley was writing – in the 1870s – a change in attitude wrought by the *Lancet* enquiry was already developing. So although his sense of entering a punitive institution is no doubt accurate, Henley was in all likelihood better off than he might have been a decade or so earlier.

The legacy of the Poor Law

The same space, then and now (opposite). Above is the outpatients' waiting hall at the London Hospital in 1876. Below, the same space has, today, been humanised and domesticated by the NHS, with revenue-generating activities in the foreground.

The *Lancet* investigation helped prompt the great infirmary building boom of the 1870s. The new infirmaries (which like St Stephen's, Fulham Road, were eventually inherited by the National Health Service) were thus the fruit of years of agitation, and their construction was originally confined to enlightened parishes. Workhouse medical officers organised themselves, and tried to improve facilities nationwide. But even as late as 1910, many Poor Law doctors – unable to afford surgical dressings from their salaries – were relying on charitable gifts of old rags for bandages.[12]

The Poor Law Board was not abolished until 1929, and the Poor Law itself only officially ceased to apply to health care in 1948. So at the time of my childhood in the 1950s, these buildings, along with all their cultural baggage, had only just been absorbed into the new National Health Service.

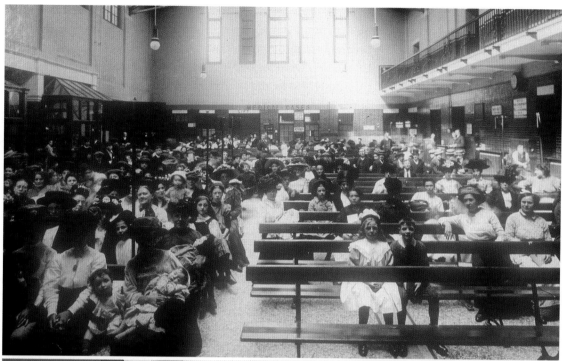

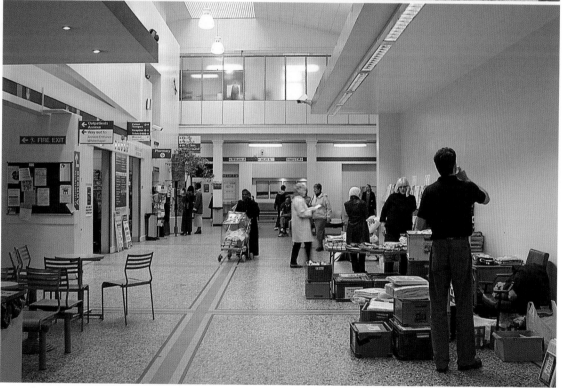

At the time of the establishment of the New Poor Law, in the 1830s, money had been found for an extensive nationwide programme to purchase land and erect purpose-made buildings for the new workhouses. The infirmary building programme of the reforming 1870s did the same. But when the National Health Service was established in the immediate aftermath of the Second World War, no money could be spared for new buildings.

Old hospital and infirmary buildings were pressed into service, bringing their characteristic ambiences with them. Old staff were employed by the new organisation, bringing older attitudes and ways of doing things with them. Although valiant attempts were made to create a new atmosphere within these old buildings, the enormous weight of previously unmet need overwhelmed the new service, and the root and branch upgrading which could have assisted was shelved for the better times everyone hoped would follow austerity. The cold hand of the past – in interpersonal relationships, attitudes, and architecture – laid a heavy weight upon the progress of the fledgling institution.

Untold smogs seemed to have left the brick facades of the old workhouse infirmaries dull and dingy, down at heel: and still daunting, too. That I and many like me absorbed the local folklore about the Knacker's Yard is hardly surprising. And despite the National Health Service, these places still felt – indeed still can sometimes feel – very much 'half-workhouse and half-jail', with a kind of inherent bleakness difficult to disguise.

Hospital design

Bird's eye view of the quadrangles of the old St Thomas's Hospital, Southwark, a century before its demolition in the 1860s to make way for London Bridge Station (opposite). Its Victorian successor, still in use, was built to a pavilion plan design on reclaimed land across the river from the Houses of Parliament.

Now, thankfully, half a century after the establishment of the National Health Service, the old buildings I have been describing are gradually being replaced or superseded. But sometimes the new buildings seem, not only to myself, unsuitable.

At a conference at the Wellcome Trust in the early 1990s, there was a discussion of so-called 'deep hospitals' (a favourite idea among architects between the 1960s and 1980s) in which Dr Aileen Adam of Addenbrooke's Hospital memorably spoke out about the disorientating effects of windowless rooms, especially in intensive care units: 'Patients go berserk, everybody goes berserk!'[13]

The therapeutic value of natural fresh air, natural light and

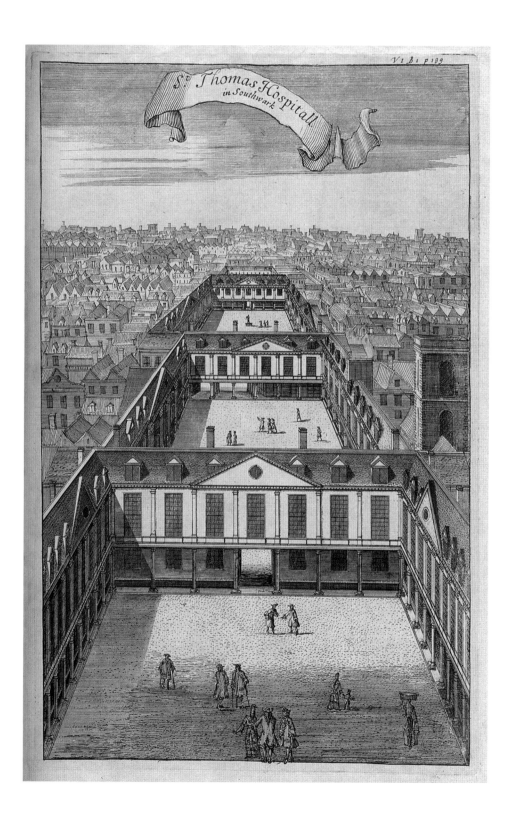

St. Thomas Hospitall in Southwark

natural landscape – particularly for bed-bound patients and sleep-deprived staff – emerged several times during discussion.

We now seem to be in the process of revisiting architectural forms of some antiquity in the healing business. The process is perhaps exemplified by the fine hospital with which this essay began, the Chelsea and Westminster, but also by others outwith the metropolis, such as the new St Mary's Hospital in the Isle of Wight, which has been designed to use half the energy of a conventional hospital, and which features lovely courtyards and natural vistas.

For centuries, the courtyard was a favourite configuration in hospital building. Some extant hospitals reach back to the era of the mediaeval cathedrals: the central courtyard at St Bartholomew's Hospital is a vestige of its ancient religious origins, and the old St Thomas's Hospital, before it left the Borough (where it was also established before the Reformation), was composed of an inter-connected series of great courtyards. Other famous hospitals erected in the eighteenth and nineteenth centuries, such as Guy's, the Foundling, and the Middlesex, utilised courtyards too.

The courtyard and the cloister are closely related, and with good reason were favoured features for country houses, as well as for Oxbridge colleges and many almshouses. In all these cases (as in monastic cloisters) the enclosed or semi-enclosed space a courtyard creates is a protected space, inward looking, concen-trated, secure, fostering privacy within a community, and yet with plenty of light, air and shelter, and a satisfying vista.

The Victorians modified the courtyard hospital into the pavilion plan, highly influential from the mid-nineteenth century on. Many pavilion-plan hospitals continued to be in use right through the twentieth century, and remain so to this day.

Although championed by Florence Nightingale and often known as 'Nightingale plan', the pavilion plan has been ascribed by Nightingale's biographer Barry Smith primarily to Isambard Kingdom Brunel, whose prefabricated hospital for the Crimean wounded, sent out to Renkioi in 1855, had 22 pavilion wards connected by covered walkways, ventilation provision, ducted heating and plumbing: 'much the best hospital in the East'.[14] George Godwin, editor of the Victorian architectural journal *The Builder*, discussed the pavilion plan ideas of Dr John Roberton of Manchester so persuasively that Miss Nightingale published

Godwin's words verbatim in her *Notes on hospitals*: the idea thereafter bore Nightingale's name.[15-17]

The main idea of the pavilion plan was to promote healing and to limit the spread of hospital infections by allowing natural light and ventilation to permeate every part of the building, and to preserve open canyons for the entry of air and light between each pavilion. The light flooded in from tall windows interspersing the beds, and natural ventilation kept wards circulated with fresh air by using the power of heated air to find its own exit in apertures near the ceiling. Photographs of Victorian pavilion wards show uniformed nurses in long bright tidy wards, often with palms or other plants thriving in the central island between the aisles.

The history of hospital design suggests that the Victorians' love of fresh air and light was sensible. Before the arrival of antisepsis and aseptic surgery, cleanliness and order cut hospital-acquired infections dramatically. Despite (or perhaps because of) our access to penicillin and other antibiotics, current levels of hospital-acquired infections are atrociously high, and I feel we could usefully examine our architecture to understand why this is so.

Personally speaking, I find modern hospitals are often airless and overheated. Even where windows can be opened, they are kept firmly closed. Overheating means that nurses habitually wear thin overalls, and because of this they not infrequently object to any fresh air as a *draught*, and justify closing windows opened by patients who want air by stating authoritatively that it will make other patients cold. Infections are thus kept within doors, circulated in air conditioning, or on the movements of what the Victorians so appropriately called 'vitiated' air, which can find no escape.

Hospital builders have thought for centuries, then, that courtyards are well-adapted to healing environments. Visiting the Middlesex Hospital to see my father after a nasty operation, only to discover him missing from the ward, I found him seated in his hospital gown and slippers, happily reading on a bench in the light and air of the lovely inner courtyard there.

The views and experiences of the *users* of hospital and clinic buildings seem to me to be crucial to future designs for healing institutions. Yet they are seldom sought. Architectural styles, like medical certainties, change over time. Now that we are at last jettisoning the old architecture of the punitive Poor Law, it is appropriate that we should be seeking to address the human needs of patients and staff, for such seems to be the lesson of the long saga of hospital and infirmary design: hospitals which centre upon green spaces for emotional and spiritual repose offer ideal environments for good care and recovery.

However, although architecture does seem important, and surely architectural forms can help, we must not place too much stress on them. It is less the architecture than the ethos of the place which is key. The old workhouse which now serves as the outpatients' department to the Middlesex Hospital in Cleveland Street had a central courtyard opening upon a green space. But the green space was the workhouse burial ground, and the courtyard was where the paupers had to beat carpets and break granite.

Acknowledgements

Thanks are due to Brian Hurwitz, to Jane Wildgoose and to Deborah Kirklin, for discussion and encouragement in the writing of this chapter.

References

1 Nightingale F. *Notes on hospitals*. London: Parker, 1859.

2 Twining L. *A letter to the President of the Poor Law Board on workhouse infirmaries*. London: Hunt, 1866.

3 Rodgers J. Workhouse into hospital: not grim enough for Russia. *Health Soc Serv J* 1982;**92**(4783):180–1.

4 Rogers J. *Reminiscences of a workhouse medical officer*. London: Fisher Unwin, 1889.

5 Longmate N. *The workhouse*. London: Croom Helm, 1974.

6 Richardson R, Hurwitz B. Joseph Rogers and the reform of workhouse medicine. *BMJ* 1989;**299**:1507–10.

7 Twining L. *Recollections of life and work*. London: Arnold, 1893.

8 Lancet Sanitary Commission for Investigating the State of the Infirmaries of Workhouses. *Report of the Commissioners on Metropolitan Infirmaries*. London: The Lancet, 1866.

9 Hart E. *An account of the condition of the infirmaries of London workhouses*. London: Chapman & Hall, 1866.

10 Anon. Workhouse reform. *BMJ* 1870;**(1)**:415–6.

11 Henley WE. *Poems*. London: Nutt, 1906.

12 Webb SB. The state and the doctor. London: Longmans, 1910. Quoted in: Crowther MA. Paupers or patients? *J Hist Med* 1984;**39**:37.

13 Personal communication from Dr Aileen Adam, Addenbrooke's Hospital, Cambridge.

14 Smith FB. *Florence Nightingale: reputation and power.* New York: St Martin's Press, 1982.

15 Taylor J. *The architect and the pavilion hospital.* London: Leicester University Press, 1997.

16 King A. Hospital planning: revised thoughts on the origin of the pavilion principle in England. *Medical History* 1966:360–73.

17 Richardson R, Thorne R. *The Builder illustrations index.* London: Institute of Historical Research, 1995.

4

'Take Art': opening the doors of the National Gallery

GHISLAINE KENYON

Gallery educator Ghislaine Kenyon describes innovations at the National Gallery which have made its works accessible to people who might not otherwise enter an art gallery: the homeless, teenage mothers, and sick children. A community cultural resource has become a source of healing. She commends similar initiatives, and calls on other guardians of the nation's cultural heritage to follow the National Gallery's lead.

The presence of the visual arts in British health care environments has a long and continuing history. But the art displayed has had many different roles, not all connected with healing. In medieval hospitals patients were encouraged to pray before images of God and the saints; for their own recovery, and for the souls of the hospital's patrons. Later, hospitals commissioned art works to impress governors and grandees rather than for the benefit of patients. Hogarth's two large paintings of New Testament stories of healing, *The pool of Bethesda* and *The good Samaritan*, which he painted for St Bartholomew's Hospital in London, were hung on a staircase never used by patients.

Twenty-first century hospitals such as London's Chelsea and Westminster Hospital take a more democratic view. In consultation with staff and patients its hospital arts trust collects art and hangs it around the institution for patients, staff and visitors to enjoy. The work, which is mainly contemporary and commissioned, and occasionally of huge scale, decorates and animates public spaces and wards. It also encourages viewers to look further, and to question and interact with it. The aim is to enhance patients' hospital experience, and to promote the enjoyment of all arts.

A recent academic research project based at the hospital has supported the wealth of anecdotal evidence supporting the role of the arts in the healing process.[1] In the Chelsea and Westminster much of the art, such as Allen Jones' gigantic sculpture *Acrobat,* is site–specific, ie designed to work within the architectural scheme. But is it only this kind of art – contemporary commissions, often cheerfully coloured, and largely 'friendly' – that can speak to patients, or can the art hanging or standing in our national and regional galleries and museums also work in this way? And is the art that decorates the hospital *only* decorative, or might there be ways of engaging with it more closely?

I want to use the case of the National Gallery in London as an example of a place and an institution of healing in the broadest sense; one that helps the individual become whole. The model we have developed at the National Gallery can be adapted to other galleries.

The National Gallery

At the National Gallery, we start with some disadvantages as far as persuading the non gallery-going public that there is something for them inside. Although we have over five million visitors annually, most of these are tourists or locals who know what they're looking for. If you ask ten random people what the National Gallery means to them, three may mention art but wouldn't care to give examples, two will shrug their shoulders, and the other five will name its Trafalgar Square location. Outside, daily, thousands of tourists take each other's photos, plunge into fountains and feed pigeons.

Only a small percentage of these people will actually enter our front doors. Until recently, our primary problem was that you couldn't even see the entrance doors from the street – let alone the exhibits inside. Prior to the pedestrianisation of Trafalgar Square, if you decided to enter you would have had to ascend the awkward staircase, pass through the neo-classical portico, ascend more stairs and then cross a solemn central hall more gentlemen's' club than art gallery (all red, leather-covered sofas and green damask wall fabric hung with 'boys'' paintings of Napoleonic battles by Vernet). Finally, you may find what you may have come for. This, of course is a mid-nineteenth century

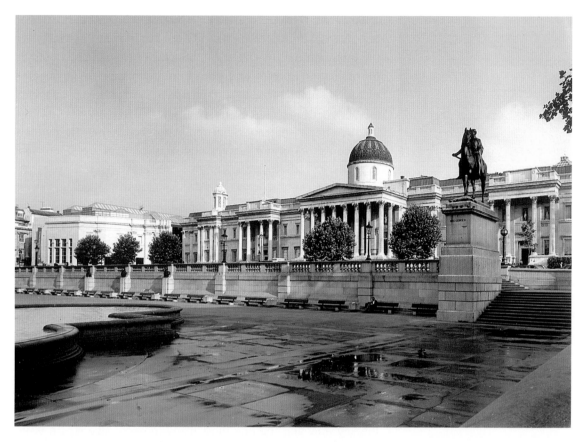

building and, like many regional galleries, was built at a time when art galleries were temples of art.

When you do find the art, what are you confronted with? A relatively small collection of paintings (no sculpture or drawings to speak of) painted between 1250 and 1900: all by dead, white, European artists, most of them male. The paintings largely depict a world of impossibly grand people, who pose for their portraits or take centre stage as heroes of ancient history or myth. This is a place where pious and remote deities and saints gaze down at you, or across you, but never meet your eyes, and distant, faded, classical landscapes stretch away from you.

Once in front of these pictures what is a visitor supposed to do? Is there an ideal amount of time to spend with a picture, which will leave the viewer feeling suitably moved? And if you don't feel moved, have you done something wrong or are you in some way inadequate? Do you even feel a bit cheated? Perhaps this isn't the place for you after all.

The grand façade of the National Gallery (1838, architect William Wilkins). The institution was intended as a 'people's gallery': the Trafalgar Square location was chosen because it was considered to be at the centre of London. The rich could drive there in their carriages from the West End; the East End poor could reach it on foot.

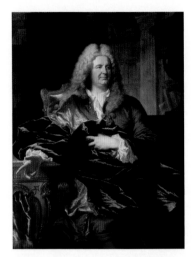

'Antoine Pâris' by Hyacinthe Rigaud (1659–1743) This type of aspirational portrait has been commissioned by the rich since the Renaissance, and is to be seen in countless country houses and galleries. Pâris was the son of an innkeeper and became a wealthy financier. Here he is painted, in court portrait-style, amid elaborate furniture and fine drapery.

Fortunately there are other ways of telling the story. The National Gallery was founded by Act of Parliament in 1824 with the intention that its collection, bought for the nation, would be for the nation to enjoy and learn from. Admission to the people's pictures would be free, a fact much admired by foreign visitors of the period. Even children were to be allowed in. This was done not for the child's edification but rather to ensure that the mothers who could not afford nursemaids would not be excluded from the gallery.

When it came to a decision about a site, Parliament opted, despite significant opposition, for a place that would be equidistant from the rich West End and the poorer sections in the east. It was to be a resource truly accessible to the whole of London's population.

The priority of provision of a democratic geographical location for the collection has been balanced in more recent times by the equally vital requirement for intellectual access to the works on display. If the subject and style of many of the works seem remote to visitors, they can be explained and interpreted in publications, labels, audio guides and websites. Guided tours can provide ready-made itineraries through the maze of rooms and artistic styles.

But there is a third type of access which is, in the end, perhaps the key one, and the one most likely to encourage return visits. This is the creation of a sense that visitors' own responses to the paintings are as valid as any curatorial commentary. Personal responses are often most easily elicited when people look at art in the company of others; when a dialogue can take place and there can be a mixture of contributions, alongside those of gallery professionals.

National Gallery Education pioneered this kind of facilitated group discussion of pictures in the 1980s with its first programme of guided tours for thirteen to eighteen year olds, led by gallery teachers. These gallery teachers are experts in their fields, but the primary aim of the tours is not to teach art history (although of course we wanted young people to leave the gallery with age-relevant knowledge of the methodologies of art history and some art historical facts). The aims of the tours are to familiarise young people with galleries in general (this is a requirement of the National Curriculum for Art) and with the National Gallery in particular, to teach or enhance visual literacy skills (how one 'reads' a picture and what questions should be asked of it) and, perhaps most importantly, to convey a sense of the enjoyment of the process of looking at pictures. One of the ways in which these aims are achieved is through an acknowledgement that there is more than one way of looking. An art historian may come to a picture armed with a large amount of contextual knowledge which she or he may use to form judgements about authorship, dating, style and technique. A lay person, however, comes to a picture with a good deal of experience of looking at the world: at people, at objects, at landscapes. In the National Gallery's collection of paintings, which is entirely pre-1900, this is also what the artists have looked at and have represented, in a more or less illusionistic manner. And so it is sometimes these shared visual experiences that first draw us to a picture.

For example, looking at Constable's *The hay wain*, comments such as 'I've seen a treetop being tossed about by the wind like that' or 'that little patch of sunlit grass is where I'd like to be', are not uncommon. Including a discussion of this aspect of looking at a picture helps a general audience to feel that they have something to contribute, and it reminds professionals that the artists who made the works were human beings who often had a particularly sensitive vision of the world, as well as the artistic skills to represent it.

The tours at the Gallery often start in this way, and to this framework of the personal bond created by unfettered looking the factual 'flesh' can be added to enrich the experience. It is up to the teachers, often influenced by the age and developmental stage of the young people, to decide how much information is presented, or when to correct a misinterpretation. As a rule, misinterpretations would only be acceptable with very young children (under seven) and after that, although speculation is vital, a conclusion would always be reached which admitted possibilities while foregrounding the known facts. A last word however: gallery teachers should always stress that, as with all learning, no one has the monopoly on information about a work, that new discoveries are constantly being made which may radically alter all previous interpretation, and that *no one* can know exactly what was in an artist's mind (sometimes not even the artist herself) when she was making the work.

We gallery educators have always been aware that, in spite of the necessary connection with formal education, 'extra-curricular' things happen on the tours. Teachers repeatedly tell us that children with learning, emotional or behavioural difficulties respond to the stimulus of paintings in a way that they, the teachers, have not encountered before. The students subsequently have better concentration, are more articulate, and are generally more engaged than usual.

Of course there are a number of factors at work here. The quality of the teaching is one: we spend considerable resources finding staff who know their art history, know the Gallery's collection, and know how to motivate reluctant teenagers or manage mercurial three-year-olds. Another factor is something in the nature of paintings; relatively large images which don't move. But the key factor seems to be the nature of the subjects represented and the skill of the artists in conveying them. Narrative paintings are usually the most popular, but we have also discovered that even where no particular narrative is implied, young people (and older people when they are 'permitted') tend to construct one anyway.

This was incidentally but incontestably proved during an exhibition we put on in 2001 curated by the artist and illustrator Quentin Blake. The exhibition was aimed at young people, though in fact two-thirds of the record 250,000 visitors were adults.

In 'Tell Me a Picture' we put up 26 pictures, mostly drawn from the National Gallery collection, but partly from other galleries with twentieth century holdings, and partly from children's book illustrations. There were two innovative elements. First, Blake's own contribution to the exhibits of large drawings on the walls of figures looking at the exhibited works. The figures were, in Blake's inimitable fashion, full of both humour and deep feeling. They had the effect of halting children's instinctive rush to get to the end, encouraging them to look and look again. The second novelty for the National Gallery was that apart from the alphabetical organising principle ('G' for Goya, 'H' for Hopper and so on) there were no words in the exhibition: the idea was for people to feel able to look at the pictures, chosen for their sense of story, without the help of information (though there was a handout provided for those who really wanted one).

The exhibition was our noisiest ever, full of people telling each other about the pictures. For people to be able to do this, they had to look at the pictures more closely, and perhaps with more

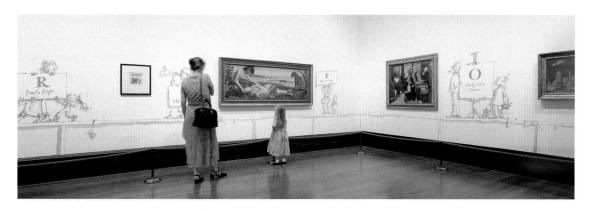

engagement than they would had information been supplied in a label or graphic panel. We also put the whole exhibition online, asking visitors to the website to respond to the works in story or poem form. We received text from over 4,500 adults and children worldwide, in ten different languages. An extraordinary and powerful involvement was often revealed, as in this submission by a Hispano-American student at a language-teaching college about the painting *The garden enclosed*, by the twentieth century artist David Jones. The artist described the work as autobiographical, saying that it showed him with his new fiancée, the then teenage Perdita Hunt. The swing and cast-away doll stand for the childhood she is about to leave behind. But the respondent seems to take in all the visual information to read the picture from a more personal point of view. The spelling, grammar and syntax are her/his own and the text is unaltered.

The 'Tell Me a Picture' exhibition, curated by illustrator Quentin Blake at the National Gallery in 2001. The exhibition had no labels or graphic panels, encouraging visitors to look for themselves, to ask questions, to speculate and so to become genuinely engaged.

> Every day at the same time and at same place this two people get together in a forest because they love each other, they have to do it like that because her parents don't let her have a boyfriend, they want her to finish the school. She love him very much, she was too young to have a boyfriend because she have to study so that way she find a good job in the future. In the farm they feel good with all the animals around them and the nature look very nice; they hope this way the time will pass? and she will be able to show her boyfriend to her parents and they will accept the relationship.

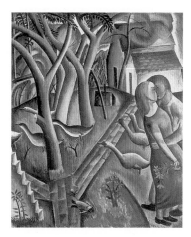

'The garden enclosed' by David Jones (1895–1974) This autobiographical work showing the artist and his teenage fiancée inspired personal responses by visitors to the 'Tell Me a Picture' website: interpretations included a student identifying with the young girl meeting her boyfriend 'secretly', and a four-year-old who said it was a farmer and his wife who so loved kissing that all their geese ran away.

Such interpretations raise fundamental questions about the way people experience visual art, a theme explored well in the philosopher John Armstrong's book, *The intimate philosophy of art*.

Armstrong reminds us that when we look at a representational image, we inevitably bring to the process visual memories of the thing or scene represented as experienced in our own lives, as well as any other representations of the subject we may have encountered. We are thus predisposed to like or dislike the work, or perhaps to pick it out from a whole wall of pictures in the first place.

> Someone who 'hardly knows the first thing about art' – in terms of specialist information – finds that the door still stands open to a fruitful encounter with individual works of art. That person already possesses, perhaps, the resources which constitute a good ground for engaging with art. A child might be struck by the red autumn leaves lying on green grass; a patch of sunlight in the distance tempts the eye and makes one feel how nice it would be to be over there; for a moment one stares intently at a wooden fence in a suburban street, absorbed in the various marks and stains which make rich an otherwise banal surface... Perceptual memories like these provide us with the material out of which we can fashion a personal relationship to a work of art. We each have our own history of impassioned looking – of looking which is woven through with feeling.[2]

On the 'Tell Me a Picture' website, the artist's explanation for the picture was not supplied alongside the image but had to be accessed via a link to another web page. Whilst I am, naturally, not arguing against the need for art historians, the decision to provide 'expert' commentary or not at this initial stage of an individual's encounter with an image is likely to have some sort of impact on the nature of that response.

The schools programme provides daily evidence of the way in which first-time visitors can experience a passionate involvement even with 'difficult' paintings, well beyond what is sometimes called art appreciation. Based on this evidence it was decided ten years ago to extend the programme to include different groups of people who might not be tempted through the gallery's doors on their own initiative, but who would perhaps not regret it if they were. The venture has progressed organically, through relationships with a number of institutions. It has proved to be of great mutual benefit in every case.

Artists without homes

The longest-established of these programmes is a project involving work with homeless artists. Our neighbour, the church of St Martin-in-the-Fields, has provided the highly regarded Social Care Unit for London's rough sleepers and others for over 50 years. As well as providing a wide range of services meeting clients' practical needs, the unit offers art, creative writing and music groups. The staff believe firmly that participating in the arts can help provide a route back to the self-esteem their clients need if they are to find the home, job and community many are seeking.

For example, a weekly, 'drop-in' taught session in an art studio offers client-artists the opportunity to make art, some of which is subsequently exhibited in an annual exhibition in the gallery at St Martin's. Around 10 years ago, staff from the National Gallery's Education Department visited the exhibition. Together with the St Martin's art tutor they decided to devise a programme of regular monthly visits to the National Gallery for users of the Social Care Unit. The visits, now an established programme, are led by Colin Wiggins from the National Gallery, himself a practising artist.

The visits allow the homeless artists to become familiar with the collection as a resource for their own work. Talks are now attended by a minimum of nine or ten regular clients, some of whom no longer need the unit's other services but have continued to use the studio, and by staff from the St Martin's unit.

What is achieved in these sessions is rich and complex. Because the clients are there as artists, rather than as homeless people, they see the visits as opportunities to develop their own professional skills in the company of other professionals. Through this group process, clients, many of whom have learning difficulties or mental illness, can also improve their social and communication skills.

Lastly, but vitally, Colin Wiggins has become aware that his choice of mainly large, narrative pictures has enabled clients to tell their own stories through their own interpretations of the paintings. A particularly powerful example is a client's reading of Titian's extraordinary late work *The death of Actaeon*. The subject is taken from Ovid's *Metamorphoses*. In revenge for surprising her as she bathed naked in the woods, the goddess Diana transformed Actaeon into a stag, causing his own hounds to attack and kill him.

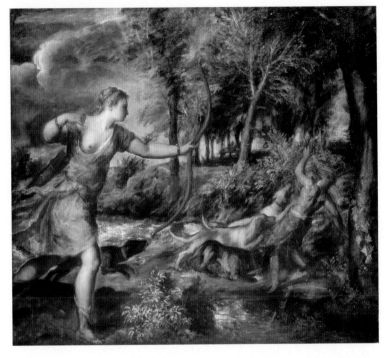

'The death of Actaeon' by Titian (about 1487–1576) A late work by the Venetian artist, which continues to fascinate viewers with its (for the date) loose painting technique, and dark subject taken from Ovid's *Metamorphoses*: the hapless Actaeon who was transformed into a stag by the goddess Diana after he surprised her as she bathed.

The picture was perceived by an elderly client as a metaphor for old age. He saw Actaeon as representing Titian himself, and the dogs as Titian's (and therefore, perhaps, his own) deteriorating faculties attacking his abilities as an artist.

This illuminating view demonstrates the conclusion that all of us who work on these programmes have reached: that the open-ended process by which visitors and gallery professionals look and interpret paintings together can be mutually enriching.

For the visitor, being able to express responses to receptive gallery professionals can be an empowering experience. From the staff's point of view such a reading, and perhaps also the practical artistic work that can result from the looking experience (so that a painting is used for the production of a further object) adds to the story of the original painting itself.

Art historians know a great deal about Titian from a great many sources, including the paintings themselves, but they do not know everything. We cannot say for certain that the ageing Titian was *not* at some possibly subconscious level expressing a frustration with old age when he painted *The death of Actaeon*. And what we can be sure about is that this particular visitor's experience of Titian at the National Gallery included both exposure to curatorial information (authorship of painting, dating and iconography) and the opportunity to propose valuable new insights or lend new meaning to a work through his own response to it.

This successful model of a cultural institution linking into existing arts provision in a social care setting is now being taken up by other museums and galleries, such as the Courtauld Institute of Art Gallery at Somerset House.

Teenage mothers

The clients of the St Martin's Social Care Unit art group are of course voluntary visitors to the gallery. Our schools programme has, however, also put us in touch with another socially excluded group who are brought to the gallery on educational trips. Teenage mothers from a Bristol unit make regular visits to the gallery as part of their art curriculum.

When they first arrive, these young women are often less than enthusiastic about the visit. Their behaviour – arms folded unco-operatively, sighing, loud remarks about the shopping in Covent Garden – inform the gallery teacher (in case she had any doubts) that the National Gallery is not the destination of choice on an otherwise desirable and rare trip to London. But an early experience with this type of group illustrates why we are convinced that it is worth attempting to persuade them otherwise.

The young mothers and a gallery teacher looked at a painting by the Italian Renaissance artist, Piero di Cosimo. *Satyr mourning over a nymph* is an example of site-specific art possibly commissioned by a wealthy family as a wedding gift to a newly married relative. Its narrow, landscape format suggests that it was once part of the furnishing of a room, perhaps set into panelling, or the backboard of a bench or chest. It shows a nymph lying on the ground in between a satyr and a dog, both of whose heads are inclined in grief over her. The nymph has wounds to her hand, wrist and throat.

The nymph is shown as a contemporary ideal of feminine beauty with rounded stomach. The story depicted is not known for certain, but it may relate to Cephalus and Procris, a tale of marital infidelity, again taken from Ovid's *Metamorphoses* in which Procris is accidentally killed by her husband Cephalus, while he is out hunting with a spear that she had given him.

The teacher had selected this painting because starting with a picture around which there is uncertainty sometimes encourages viewers to contribute more confidently and imaginatively to a discussion. But before the teacher had even had a chance to introduce the painting, a young pregnant woman who, five minutes before, had been the most sullen of the protesters, and two minutes before had been texting her boyfriend, suddenly put down her phone. 'She's pregnant' (interested, though arms still firmly folded) 'and I know what this story is – she's fallen pregnant and her dad's punished her, and now she's dead'. This statement seemed to resonate with the rest of the group, who began to freely offer their own suggestions. They searched the painting for clues, agreeing and disagreeing over interpretation or identifications, constructing meaning for themselves. A mature discussion had taken place, and the group was keen to see more.

The point about this anecdote is that the communicative quality of the painting alone had the power to inspire speculation and discussion. The starting point for the students, though, was clearly an identification with the subject that the teachers had not predicted. The narratives that emerged were, though mediated through a shared image and at a safe distance from their narrators and from their audience, without doubt in some measure personal. These narratives took on a universal character, and became even more powerful. The young mothers' teachers confessed to us later that they had not expected these reactions. They were impressed by the young women's confidence in expressing themselves in potentially alienating public spaces, before the kind of art which was (on the face of it) altogether unfamiliar and remote.

'Satyr mourning over a nymph' by Piero di Cosimo (about 1462 – after 1515) Another mythological subject, the precise story unknown though; viewers are, however, unfailingly attracted by the half-bestial satyr's deeply human response to the nymph's plight, and by the mysterious blue landscape where strange animals play, oblivious to the tragedy in the foreground.

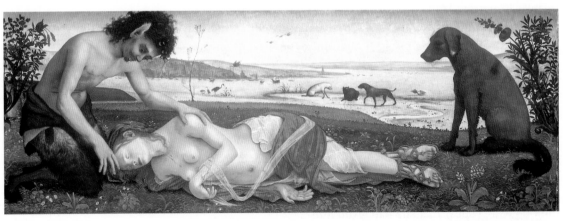

'Take Art'

'Take Art' is a three-year-old project in which the gallery works with young patients and staff in fourteen hospitals in the London area. 'Take Art' grew from an existing relationship we had with the local Great Ormond Street Children's Hospital. Mobile patients visited the gallery with a teacher from the hospital school, as part of a programme of regular school trips to various venues. Funding was found to bring the gallery to the hospital after the teacher suggested that bed- or hospital-bound patients might benefit from these experiences.

The project fits most naturally into our schools programme, with bed- and hospital-bound young people entitled to pursue their education in the best sense of the word. Security issues preclude the use of originals, and any reproductions must be wipeable, so that they can be used by barrier-nursed patients, and small enough to use for bedside teaching. High-quality, A1-sized, laminated prints are therefore used.

A number of existing gallery teachers with experience in special needs teaching have engaged with this project operating in fourteen of the hospitals in the London area with hospital schools or teaching units. They attend training provided by the Chelsea and Westminster Hospital School, which specifically addresses the ethical, legal and practical issues of working in a hospital setting.

The images are chosen to support the curriculum. For example, a still life can provide a resource for students tackling that part of the art curriculum, an altarpiece showing the story of the Magi can be used for religious education.

Sometimes the looking session is followed up by a practical one which might be art-based, but could just as well be a literacy exercise. Each session is fully discussed with the teacher, and sometimes also clinical staff, beforehand. The situations in which we work vary considerably and we need to be flexible: some hospital schools have large purpose-built school rooms, others use dedicated corners of wards, and in some much of the teaching has to be done by the bedside.

When we work with seriously ill patients we may be gowned and masked in private rooms. We also visit secure psychiatric units. The patients may be anything from four to seventeen years old and the size of the groups may change from minute to minute as patients leave for, and return from, treatment or tests. For this reason, and because we only visit twice a term, the prints, together with teaching notes containing basic information about the pictures and the artists and suggestions for using them in lessons, are left behind at the hospitals. They become permanent resources for hospital teachers to use as and when they wish. At first we envisaged that this would be in the context of lessons, but we have learned that, as with the young mothers, the outcomes of the visits are never predictable.

Some encounters between patients, pictures and gallery teachers echo those that took place in the gallery with the artists without homes and the young mothers, but in a sense take things a step further. The following examples are of course anecdotal, unmeasurable in any scientific sense, other than that they are instances of events which recur and recur. All client's names have been altered.

Soraya and Piero di Cosimo

A gallery teacher from the team had been working for several months with an 11-year-old leukaemia patient, Soraya, who had come to London from another country for treatment. Over that period Soraya was in and out of remission. Both her parents were health care professionals, but (or maybe therefore) in denial of her illness, which made the situation a particularly painful one. The hospital teachers had identified her enthusiasm for drawing and painting, and thought she might enjoy looking at pictures as well. That she did was clear at the first visit, when Soraya asked to keep one of the prints in her room. She chose a Renaissance painting of the Annunciation. Soraya was a Muslim and not familiar with this story from the Christian tradition, but she became attached to the picture, loving the patterns and colours and the graceful figure of the Virgin Mary. The gallery teacher built up a good relationship with Soraya, bringing several different images at each visit. This often seemed to relieve her periods of sadness and fear.

At a certain point, when the leukaemia had returned very virulently, the teacher and clinical staff suggested that the Piero di Cosimo might be a suitable image to offer Soraya. The reasoning here was twofold: first, the picture fitted into the students' curriculum on Greek mythology; and second, the teacher felt that the picture might enable her to express, while discussing the story, some of her own feelings. It should be pointed out that we always ask patients if they are happy to look at the image – if a patient has a negative reaction we offer something different.

However this was not the case with Soraya on this occasion. She asked if she could keep it; she thought it was peaceful and beautiful. A few days later a nurse came into her room and asked her why she had such a depressing picture. Here Soraya became the vulnerable, compliant child patient and agreed to have the nurse take it down from the wall. However, when the gallery teacher returned on the following visit (which turned out to be the last), the *Satyr mourning over a nymph* was back up on the wall, where Soraya had, significantly, asked her mother to replace it.

Soraya did not live for much longer, but the feeling on the ward was that this picture, with what many people describe as its sense of acceptance, may have helped her in some way to face her death with less fear.

Which pictures are selected for use in hospitals is an important issue. The National Gallery's paintings are often very serious, sometimes violent, and only rarely involve bright colours. Is there a right kind of image that patients in hospital need, or should look at? Are some images unsuitable?

Some research into these questions has been conducted by Roger Ulrich of Texas A&M University,[3] involving a group of patients recovering from major heart surgery. The question of which type of image put up in a patient's room speeded recovery was asked. Measurements of physiological responses such as blood pressure and requirements for analgesia were taken, and it was found that, perhaps unsurprisingly, most patients preferred photographs of lakes and forests to abstract expressionist paintings.

Whilst Ulrich's study involved patients' recovery from acute major surgery, our work is with patients confronting the rather different challenges of chronic illness and, often, protracted and monotonous hospitalisation. The prints we use in this educational setting are those which seem to be of value in addressing feelings of isolation, fear or anxiety, feelings which are experienced all too often by young people who are in hospital because of physical or mental illness.

We have found few images that do not seem to trigger some interest and discussion. Most hospital teachers and clinical staff tell us that we should *not* avoid using images that deal with mortality or unhappiness. We have found that patients presented with ostensibly happy or neutral works often read their own preoccupations with mortality or unhappiness into them.

The nurse and Joseph Wright of Derby's Experiment

Another story illustrates how 'Take Art' can help children to express ideas and feelings, and provide staff with important new insights.

When Tim was eight years old his illness required frequent dialysis. A gallery teacher visited him on the busy dialysis ward, and showed him this picture by Joseph Wright of Derby. *An experiment on a bird in the air pump* is an eighteenth century portrayal of a scientific demonstration of the efficacy of a then relatively newly-invented piece of equipment, the air pump. A white cockatiel has been placed inside a glass receiver and the air pump is being used to create a vacuum.

The bird will die if the demonstrator continues to deprive it of air. Wright leaves us in doubt as to whether or not the cockatoo will be reprieved. There are a wide range of individual reactions to the experiment, from the anxious children and the excited young men on the left, to the pensive old man on the right and the slightly ambiguous responses of the young couple on the left – is the woman more engrossed in her man than in the experiment, and is he gazing back at her or *past* her to get a better view of the science?

Tim was fascinated with the image, and spotted the bird in the container immediately (most visitors looking at this picture notice the young girls first). His reading of the painting was also unusual: he said that he saw a bird and all around it people trying to make it better. He interpreted the air pump as a kind of dialysis machine. The teacher expressed interest at this reading but went on to explain the notion of the pump because Tim was also fascinated by the science. (It is worth repeating that although, as gallery teachers, we cannot deliver misinformation about our pictures, sometimes – particularly with young children – it is appropriate to leave an interpretation 'hanging'. The teacher's comment might be: 'It does look as if that might be happening'.)

'Take Art' sessions are often observed informally by the hospital's teaching or clinical staff, and in this case a nurse stopped to listen. Afterwards she told the gallery teacher that she had learned a great

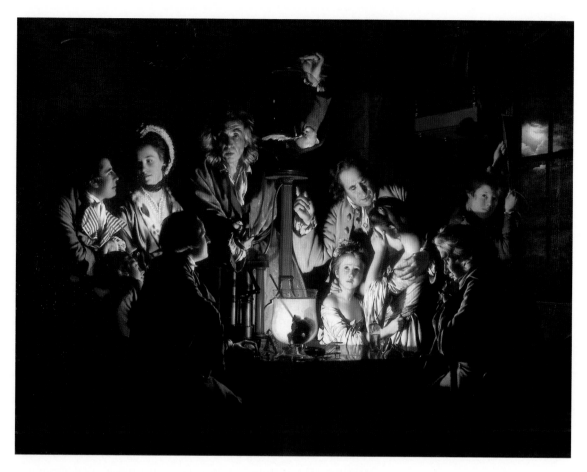

deal during the session, not so much about Wright of Derby and his painting (although she had); instead, she said, listening to Tim talking about the picture had given her an insight into how he was feeling. She remarked that she spent so much time on the ward plugging children into and out of machines that the mechanics of the situation had completely taken over; she had forgotten about the children attached to them. The teacher felt that the way this intervention had prompted the nurse to look at her own work situation alone made it worthwhile, quite apart from what happened to Tim.

'An experiment on a bird in the air pump' by Joseph Wright of Derby (1734-1797) This work illustrates the artist's own fascination with science: the central figure demonstrates an air-pump by withdrawing air from a container holding a now-suffering cockatiel. Patients often identify with this bird, seeing it as a centre of attention but also as trapped and sick.

Meaning and making

The final examples from the 'Take Art' story relate to the creation of further objects as the result of a looking session.

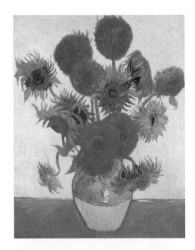

'Sunflowers' by Van Gogh (1853–1890) Artists' biographies are not usually the main focus of 'Take Art' sessions, but it's hard to separate Van Gogh's well-documented final struggle with mental illness from his expressive late works. This was one of a series painted in an optimistic period while Van Gogh waited in Arles for the arrival of fellow artist Gauguin.

A terminally ill nine-year-old looked at Van Gogh's *Sunflowers* as part of a topic on the artist. He loved the picture but also became involved in the story behind it. Van Gogh originally painted this and other versions of his vases of sunflowers to decorate a room in his house for his fellow painter Gauguin. Van Gogh had invited him to stay in a bid to establish an artists' colony in the southern French town of Arles. Although the invitation was well intentioned, Van Gogh and Gauguin had a famous falling out; the quarrel ended with Gauguin's abrupt return to Paris and Van Gogh's severing of part of his ear in despair. This act was a symptom of the mental illness which eventually drove the artist to suicide.

Although the teacher did not describe the final incidents in Van Gogh's life, the boy listened with interest when she explained how Van Gogh had, when in the asylum at nearby St Rémy, found comfort in painting; in particular the boy liked the idea of Van Gogh painting views of the world outside and bringing these back into the hospital, so that the beautiful and lively world outside would be near him when he was shut away inside. Whether it was this notion of painting as a source of comfort, or maybe the theme of room decoration, which inspired the boy, he decided to decorate his own room by painting a frieze of sunflowers, spending a great deal of time and energy on the project.

On another occasion, a group of cancer patients in early adolescence had been looking at *Tobias and the angel* by the Verrocchio workshop. The picture shows a moment from an Old Testament story, in which the boy Tobias is accompanied on a long journey by the Archangel Raphael. The students were drawn to the idea of guardian angels, and began making their own imaginative versions. One of the group, an 11-year-old girl, died during this period. The remaining students spontaneously decided to make one for her, decorating the frame with objects symbolising the girl's favourite things such as sweet wrappers and figures cut from CD covers. This picture was hung in the hospital schoolroom as a memorial to their dead friend. Their teacher commented that the activity had enabled the students to express their grief for their friend, and also for themselves. At the same time it consoled them, because it was such a positive and creative act.

'Tobias and the angel' by the Verrocchio (1437–1488) workshop The subject of this work is from the Bible. Its theme is the healing of blind Tobit by his son Tobias. Patients find this a comforting image, perhaps because of the trust the young boy seems to place in his angelic guide as they travel through the stony landscape.

Fifteen-year-old Jason attends the psychiatric unit of a London hospital and lives with his severely psychotic mother, many of whose problems he seems to have adopted as his own. In a session

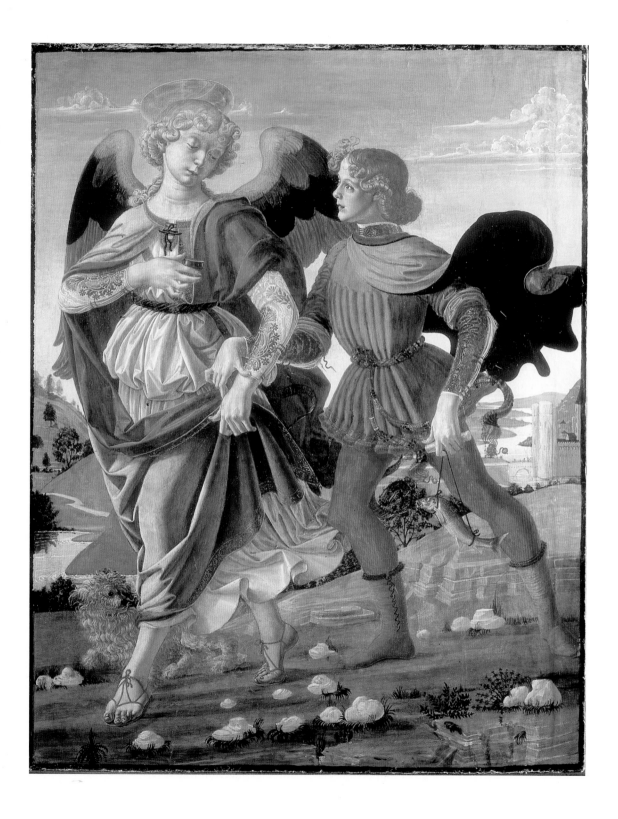

during which the students looked at Gossaert's *Adoration of the Kings*, Jason contributed nothing to the discussion but asked if he could make a picture. Over the next few weeks he spent many hours on a large drawing in coloured pencil, in which he had taken the Gossaert and subtly transformed it: the central figure of the Virgin Mary is visibly weeping and instead of a baby she holds a star. Jason was not able to explain his picture, but it meant a great deal to him. His teachers said he had never been interested in art before, but that subsequently he started to make other 'transcriptions' of the prints that were up in the classroom. Now Jason says he would like to go to art school.

Another student at this unit who arrived with a reputation for disruptive behaviour was involved in a session where students looked at a painting of *Saint Michael and the Devil* by the fifteenth century Spanish artist, Bermejo. The teachers in the unit wrote back to us describing the outcome of the visit:

> It has been a real turning point for the young man who was so moved by the painting and articulate and knowledgeable about the mythology surrounding it. We had absolutely no idea that this young man was interested in art, or anything else for that matter. Previously all we had seen of him in the classroom was abusive behaviour and all school reports indicated that he had moderate learning difficulties. This information will be very valuable for the medical team at ——.
>
> You may have noted that we were all astounded by his contributions to your session. This also had a strong influence on the other young people and we were able to see a much softer emotional side of him. For the young man he has gained status among his peers and we now have a route to engage him in the classroom through the history of art, because he has not been able to express himself through drawing.

Perhaps this response also says something about those of us who work with students, patients or student-patients. We often know very little about the interior world of the people in our care; about what engages them at a deep level, where engagement may often be a key to progress in mental/physical state. The pictures held in galleries around the country can provide people with an opportunity to become engaged in this way.

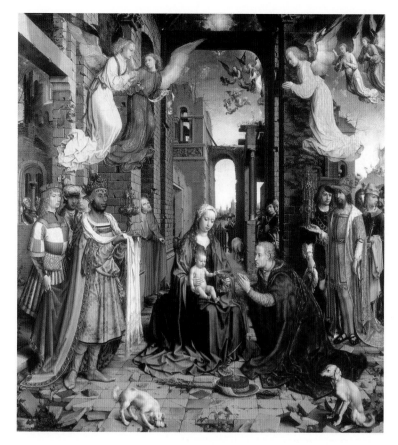

'The adoration of the Kings' by Gossaert (1503–1532) This large altarpiece painted with luscious detail includes a possible self-portait of the artist as a barely visible onlooker in the doorway to the left of Mary's head. A young psychiatric patient took the autobiographical idea in his own transcription of this work in which he appears as a star on Mary's lap.

Conclusion

The schemes described in this chapter, developed in response to specific educational needs, have evolved in directions far more wide-reaching than was originally envisaged. The gallery staff have learnt as much as any of our clients by using the gallery's resources in this way. We have been reminded of the great power possessed by the pictures we work with every day.

The artists who painted these pictures were often extraordinary people, possessed of great sensitivity. Whilst the technical skills they developed to communicate their vision of the world are an important aspect of what people notice when they look at a painting, this only partially explains the impact these works have on those who encounter them. For patients in hospital, or other groups of people with particular emotional and/or physical needs, it seems to be the content – the subjects depicted and the way they are depicted – that speaks most insistently. People in these situations seem instinctively to use the paintings as mirrors, sometimes distant or even distorted ones, of their own experiences. The fact that these experiences can exist outside themselves appears to bring comfort.

Of course, the context needs to be right: the right room, the right number in the group, the right person leading the session, and so on. For the looking activity there needs to be the right amount of time and space and conversation. Participants (including the leader) also need to feel that there is nothing that *cannot* be said about a work even when that might mean a negative response to something admired and respected by others. When all these conditions exist it is our experience that the outcomes are very positive. This reinforces our belief that looking at art makes you feel better, even when you're not ill.

References

1   Lelchuck Staricoff R, Duncan J, Wright M, Loppert S, Scott J. A study of the effects of the visual and performing arts in healthcare. *Hospital Development* 2001;**32**:25–8.
2   Armstrong J. *The intimate philosophy of art*. London: Allen Lane. 2000.
3   Ulrich R. View through a window may influence recovery from surgery. *Science* 1984;**224**(4647):420–1.

5

Integrating the arts into health care: can we affect clinical outcomes?

ROSALIA STARICOFF & SUSAN LOPPERT

Scientist Dr Rosalia Staricoff, Director of the Chelsea and Westminster Hospital Arts Research Project, and art historian Susan Loppert, Director of Chelsea and Westminster Hospital Arts, describe the results of their pioneering research at the hospital aimed at assessing the clinical impact of a vibrant hospital arts programme. Their findings counter the notion that benefits resulting from the arts in hospital environments are impossible to measure.

Introduction

In a 1997 issue of *The Lancet*, Pryle Behrman expressed the long-held belief that 'it is difficult to provide rigorous proof of the positive effects of the arts on patients' health. There are too many variables to do a trial that is statistically reliable'.[1] We challenge this assumption by describing a study at Chelsea and Westminster Hospital which uses rigorous scientific methodology to evaluate the effects of integrating the arts into health care. The main aim of this research was to provide answers to the fundamental question of whether the arts can play a meaningful role in the practice of medicine.

In this chapter we outline the quantitative results of the survey on the attitudes of patients, staff and visitors to the use of visual and performing arts at the hospital, and report on staff assessments of the extent to which the hospital's arts in health programme has influenced their desire to work there. A number of research protocols are described, carried out in different clinical units and aimed at finding out whether arts in health can play a therapeutic role by influencing parameters of clinical significance. With interest in the arts in health increasing worldwide, the need to quantify and evaluate effects has become ever more pressing.

Background

Chelsea and Westminster Hospital, London's newest NHS teaching hospital, opened in 1993. A pioneering approach of commissioning site-specific works of art while the hospital was being planned meant that the arts complemented, rather than merely adorned, innovative architectural design. Such integration of the visual arts in a hospital is unique in Britain to two hospitals designed by architects new to the design of hospitals: St Mary's, Isle of Wight (1991), and Chelsea and Westminster. As a result, patients, staff and visitors at Chelsea and Westminster are immediately welcomed by Sian Tucker's rainbow-coloured mobile *Falling leaves* tumbling five storeys, Patrick Heron's ravishing, 50 foot silk banners, and the largest indoor hospital sculpture in the world, Allen Jones' 60 foot high green, yellow and red corten steel *Acrobat*.

Chelsea and Westminster Hospital Arts, a project entirely funded by private donations, has been working within the hospital since its conception and provides all the visual arts in public areas, clinics and wards, as well as live performances each week. Hospital Arts has staged the world's first music festivals and operas in a hospital. Patients, visitors, staff, and members of the local community attend these performances, all of which are free of charge. The eclectic programme won Hospital Arts a place amongst the six finalists for the National Art Collections Fund Prize in 1996 and a citation for 'its innovative and imaginative approach to hospital healthcare which enhances the experience of patients, staff and visitors'.[2] In 2000, Hospital Arts' director won a Creative Britons Award – Britain's largest arts prize – of £20,000 for her pioneering work at the hospital, and a month later was invited to address a specially convened meeting of the parliamentary Arts and Heritage Committee at the House of Lords, an indication of the growing awareness of the importance of the arts in health care.

The question of whether the arts can play a meaningful role in health care concerns a wide range of professionals – architects, artists, medical staff, administrators and those who work for health authorities. The answers, however, have hitherto largely been based on anecdotal information or opinion-based surveys.[3]

The iconic *Acrobat* by Allen Jones (opposite) is one of three large works commissioned by Chelsea and Westminster Hospital Arts while the hospital was planned and installed during construction. It is a structure of painted corten steel and is over 60 feet high. The other two works (both overleaf) are Sian Tucker's, 75 feet high *Falling leaves*, a mobile consisting of 90 individual elements, each individually pivoted, and the three appliquéd Habotai silk banners (1993–1994) designed by Patrick Heron (1920–1999) and made by Cathy Merrow-Smith. The largest is 56 feet long, the smallest 34 feet.

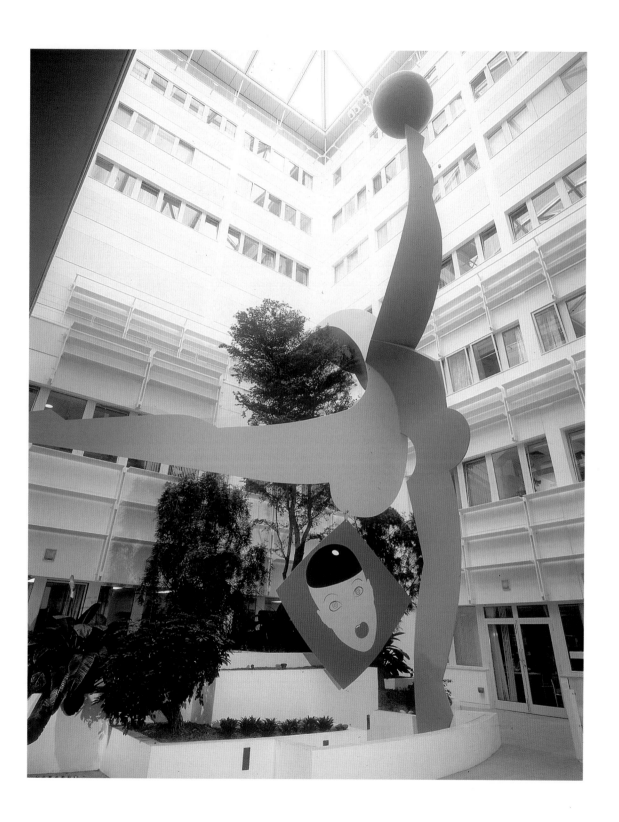

65

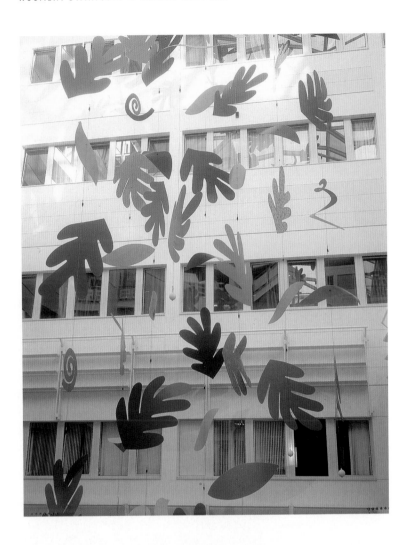

'Falling leaves' by Sian Tucker (1958–) 1993, mixed media, painted Foamex panels, stainless steel rigging and movement mechanisms.

The need for a rigorous evaluation of the effects of the arts in health care is widely recognised and the Chelsea and Westminster provides an ideal setting for such an evaluative process.

The emotional component of patients' illnesses can easily be overlooked given the pressure of work in busy hospital clinics. It is widely acknowledged that anxiety and depressive states may cause somatic symptoms, or that they may be a consequence of illness or treatment, but either way they often remain largely undetected in conventional hospital environments.[4] Physicians concerned with these issues, however, have found that the arts can fulfil a dual role: helping to detect states of depression and anxiety in their patients, and acting as a therapeutic tool.[5]

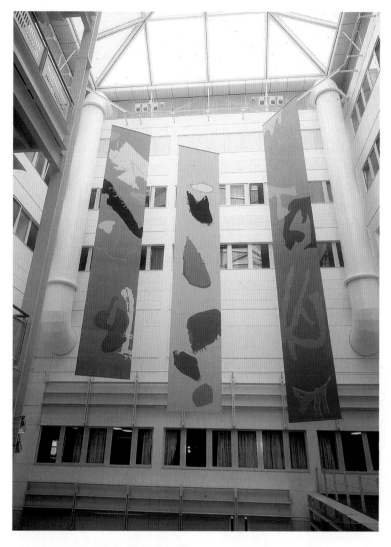

Patrick Heron's and Cathy Merrow-Smith's three appliquéd Habotai silk banners.

There have already been numerous opinion-based surveys and evaluations of arts projects. Malcolm Miles published a survey of arts projects in the NHS in 1994,[6] describing the study as qualitative rather than quantitative. He recognised that measuring the benefits for patients and staff was another question which required further research. A recent opinion-based survey conducted at the Royal Devon and Exeter Hospital found that the majority of clinical staff considered the arts to have a positive effect on patient morale.[3]

A basic overview of methods and approaches surveys of those involved in community health projects was commissioned by the

Department of Health.[7] The University of Sheffield, in association with NHS Estates and other NHS Trusts, has evaluated the effects of other aspects, such as the architectural environment and its influence on patient health outcomes, for example in accelerating recovery.[8]

Extensive research covers music in health care, including an evaluation of the effects of music in a health care project.[9] Sharon Olson has confirmed the benefits of bringing live performances to the bedside[10] and Judith Wilkinson, in her recently published evaluation of music in health care, highlights its power to '[enhance] the quality of life'.[11] In many cases patients are introduced to new art forms. An elderly patient in a wheelchair, after attending an opera on the stage at Chelsea and Westminster Hospital, said: 'I wish I could live long enough to go again to the opera; this is my first experience and it's wonderful'.

There are clear signs that the importance of the arts in health care is being recognised – for example NHS Estates now recommends that at least 1% of the cost of new capital builds be

On the stage, a large open area on the second floor of the main atrium, the Opera Project – opera company in residence since 1998 – perform Mozart's *The magic flute*. Operas staged since 1997 include Puccini's *La Bohème* and Verdi's *La Traviata*, proving that the subject of death and dying can be broached by hospital arts programmes.

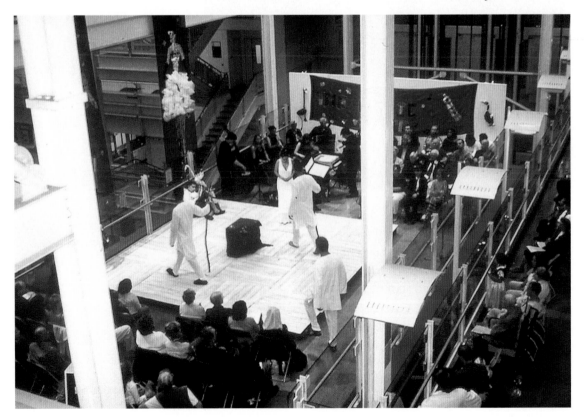

allocated to decorative enhancement of buildings. This is not mandatory, however, and more high-quality research evidence is needed if those responsible for new buildings are to be persuaded, and a new culture to accommodate twenty-first century concepts in health care environments is to be created.[12]

The challenges of working in a clinical setting

It was an enormous task to structure a research project which by the very nature of its aims and objectives had to bridge the activities of Chelsea and Westminster Hospital Arts and the health care environment without interfering with hospital routine: extensive consultation was necessary. The project needed to gain the support of medical and nursing staff, as well as managers, to conduct research in the chosen areas of the hospital. This was achieved by developing a clearly defined protocol with well-defined objectives, and ensuring the understanding and collaboration of all staff. It was essential to identify the measurements that were of clinical significance in a selected medical unit, and adapting to the routine of the clinic and not imposing any extra burden upon staff was considered to be of paramount importance. The implementation of each protocol in the selected area of research also required prior approval from the hospital's Ethics Committee, which was asked to authorise the retrieval of data from patients' notes after they had received treatment in the presence or absence of visual or performing arts.

Research methodology

1. Patient, staff and visitor attitudes to the use of the visual and performing arts in a health care setting

Evaluation forms were distributed to patients, staff and visitors in wards, where works of art are permanently displayed, in public areas, and during the course of live performances. Respondents were invited to score questions on the impact of the visual arts and performing arts on them, the value they placed on the work of Chelsea and Westminster Hospital Arts, and their opinions on the importance of the arts in the healing process. Each question was scored on a scale of one to ten; low scores were considered to represent a very low effect or none at all, and high scores of seven or more to show a positive or very positive response.

Data were collected over one year (1999/2000); more than a thousand questionnaires were completed. Responses elicited by the permanent displays of contemporary art, and a year-long programme of weekly, sometimes daily, live performances – which included classical music, jazz, world music, opera, dance, theatre, poetry and readings by writers and actors – were collated. The three populations cooperated willingly, in confidence and with anonymity.

2. The impact of an active hospital arts programme on staff recruitment and retention

Using a form modified from the patient questionnaire described above, medical, nursing, scientific, managerial and administrative staff were asked whether the integration of architecture, light, colour, works of art and live performances in the working environment would influence their decision to stay in their current work, or to apply for a job at Chelsea and Westminster Hospital. Respondents were also asked whether they would prefer to work in a modern or a traditional NHS hospital.

The questionnaire was included in the payslips of 2,200 members of staff. There were 325 respondents, among them 62 doctors, 129 nurses, 12 scientists, 20 managers and 102 administrators.

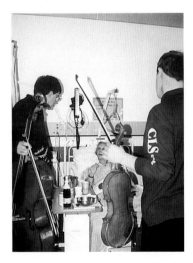

Nick Ward, and members of the City of London Sinfonia, orchestra in residence for four years, entertain patients, staff and visitors in a ward (below and opposite). Each month a quartet of or quintet of players gave an informal public concert in the mall, followed by participative workshops in wards.

3. Assessing whether arts in health can affect clinical outcomes

A customised protocol for measuring clinical outcomes was needed for each clinical unit selected for the study. A thorough review of the literature with the latest medical findings relating to our areas of research allowed the identification of physiological and biological outcomes clinically relevant for the patients taking part in the study. It was clearly important to choose outcomes appropriate to the way in which each particular unit organised both patient management and ward routine.

All protocols were designed to minimise bias which might undermine the validity of the evidence. The control group was defined as the population tested in the absence of works of art and/or live music provided by Hospital Arts. The intervention group was that population tested in the presence of the visual arts and/or live music. The same place, time of week, procedure, and medical team were used for both groups.

a. Patients receiving chemotherapy

The medical day unit for patients receiving chemotherapy was selected as an area for our research after meetings with its medical staff. We evaluated the activities of Chelsea and Westminster Hospital Arts within the clinic, rotating pictures with different themes weekly and organising various types of performance by professional musicians. After four months, a hundred examples of Zigmond and Snaith's internationally accepted 'Hospital Anxiety and Depression Scale' had been completed by patients.

Research was carried out at the same time on the same day of the week over a period of six months. We established three groups:

▷ the control group formed by patients receiving treatment in the absence of the visual arts or live music (the first two months);

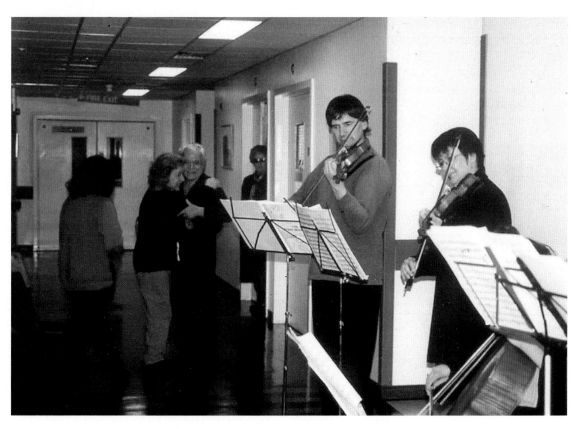

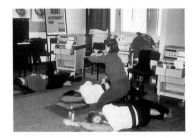

Expectant mothers in an antenatal class have their babies' foetal heartbeats measured by the cardiotochograph in the absence, and presence, of live music.

▷ the trial group (music) which consisted of patients treated in the presence of an hour of live music (the following two months); and,

▷ the trial group (visual art), those patients treated in the presence of works of art within the room (the final two months). This display was changed weekly and included landscapes, abstract work and portraits.

b. Anxiety and depression levels in pregnant women

For the expectant mother, pregnancy can bring with it not only joy but anxiety and, sometimes, depression. We therefore designed a protocol to detect and follow any changes in anxiety and depression in a group of mothers attending specific antenatal classes. They were offered an hour or an hour-and-a-half of relaxation and breathing using the Alexander Technique, under the supervision of a professional dancer. The Zigmond and Snaith scales for measuring levels of anxiety and depression were used again. Participating mothers completed the tests for anxiety and depression on arrival at the class and before leaving.

c. Antenatal patients with high blood pressure

We assessed the blood pressure – routinely taken by medical staff – of pregnant women attending the antenatal high-risk clinic, after waiting for their clinic appointment either in the absence of live music (control group), or in the presence of one hour of live music (trial group).

The day for conducting research in this area, selected following meetings with the medical staff, was the time the clinic saw pregnant women under treatment for high blood pressure. Systolic and diastolic levels of 34 women in the control group and 54 in the trial group were collected and analysed statistically.

d. The effect of live music on mothers and their unborn children

Women beyond thirty weeks of pregnancy were invited to attend live concerts performed by one or two musicians. The programme consisted of classical, jazz and pop music with the piano, violin, flute, clarinet or harp most often featured. The choice of music and type of instrument were carefully considered. The intention was to create a calming, cheerful and pleasant environment. The measurements chosen for evaluating the effect of live music were

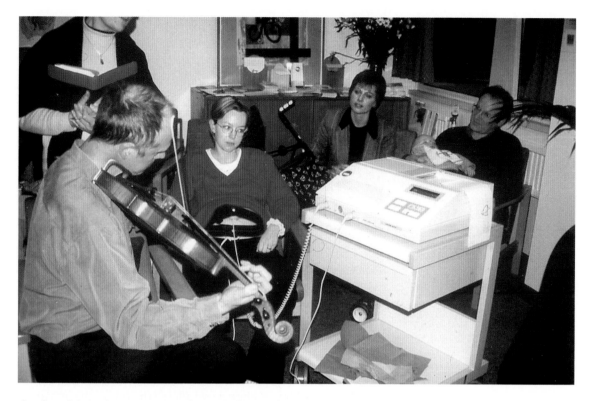

the foetal heartbeat (measured using the cardiotocograph (CTG)) and the heart rate of the mother. Both measurements were taken when the mother was resting, either with or without live music playing. All data was interpreted in collaboration with midwives and then analysed statistically.

For the first 20 minutes after the pregnant woman was connected to the CTG, the foetal heartbeat, in the absence of live music, was recorded. This provided control data for comparison with the heartbeat tracing recorded in the subsequent 20 minutes, this time in the presence of live music. Twenty five pregnant women participated in this study.

Results

1. Patient, staff and visitor attitudes to the use of the visual and performing arts in a health care setting

Quantitative analysis of the questionnaire data showed that 75% of respondents in each group (patients, staff and visitors) reported an overwhelmingly positive attitude towards the visual arts and live

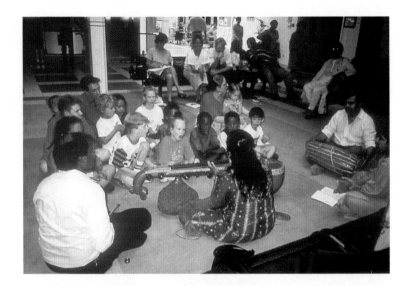

The London Veena Group giving a lunchtime concert in the busy ground floor mall. Music, theatre, dance, storytelling and puppetry are provided each week for patients, staff and visitors in wards and public areas.

performances in terms of enjoyment, stress levels, welcome distraction from immediate worries and mood enhancement.[13] Interestingly, the results suggest that in general female patients value the use of the arts in a hospital more than male patients. In addition to valuing the work of Chelsea and Westminster Hospital Arts, two-thirds of each population considered the role of the arts in the healing process to be an important one.

Statistical analysis of the questionnaires has shown that patients find live performances significantly more effective than the visual arts in helping to take their minds off immediate worries or medical problems. This finding suggests a potential therapeutic role for the arts in providing distraction from anxieties and diminishing stress levels. This would clearly benefit patients and visitors, humanising and adding value to hospital services. The results of this first year of research are published in the journal *Hospital Development*.[13]

2. The impact of an active hospital arts programme on staff recruitment and retention

The results suggest that an arts in health programme does play a part in staff decisions about where they choose to work and whether they plan to stay in post. Median scores in each group were located in the middle of the scale, indicating that staff are concerned about their working environment. Staff also indicated a clear preference for working in modern hospitals. This quantitative analysis underpins the current interest of health authorities and architects[14] in designing buildings in which the paramount importance of integrating the arts into the design of health care buildings is recognised as essential to the well-being of all those people who use these spaces.[8]

3. Assessing whether arts in health can affect clinical outcomes

a. Patients receiving chemotherapy
Anxiety levels were 20% lower than controls in patients exposed to the visual arts, and 32% lower in patients exposed to live music. Depression levels were 34% lower than controls in patients exposed to visual arts, and 31% lower for patients exposed to live music. These results provide qualitative evidence of the therapeutic benefits of integrating the arts into health care environments.

The anxiety scale was completed by 57 patients and the depression scale by 56. Regression analysis determined whether scores varied in the three groups. The scores of the trial groups were compared to those of the control group. Anxiety scores in the visual arts group were 18% lower than the scores in the control group (95% confidence interval: 47% lower to 26% higher). This result was not statistically significant ($p = 0.36$). Anxiety scores in the music group were 32% lower ($p = 0.13$).

Depression scores in the visual arts group were 34% lower ($p = 0.08$), and in the music group 31% lower ($p = 0.18$), than scores in the control group. The small size of the sample made it impossible to detect significant differences.

b. Anxiety and depression levels in pregnant women
The results demonstrated a significant reduction in levels of anxiety and depression for those mothers who took part in the relaxation class, providing evidence to support the introduction of such classes as a routine aspect of patient management.

Recorded data correspond to 77 pregnant women (90% of total participants in 10 classes). Wilcoxon matched-pairs signed-rank sum tests were used to determine whether there were changes to anxiety and depression scores following participation in the class. Anxiety scores were lower after the class – median difference in score was 1.5 (95% confidence intervals: 1 to 2) and significantly different $p < 0.001$. Depression scores were also significantly lower after the class – the median difference was 1 unit (95% confidence intervals: 0 to 1), $p = 0.003$.

c. Antenatal patients with high blood pressure

Our results showed that the women who listened to music in the waiting room tended to have lower blood pressure measurements in the clinic that followed their wait than mothers in the control group who were not exposed to live music. (It is not known whether this improvement is sustained beyond the time spent at the clinic.) An hour of live classical music with one or two musicians was provided; the harp was apparently most effective.

This was a pilot study with 34 patients in the control group and 54 in the study group. Systolic blood pressure was 3.5 mmHg lower in the study group (95% confidence interval 9.8 mmHg lower to 2.9 mmHg higher), $p = 0.28$. Diastolic blood pressure was 2.3 mmHg lower in the study group (95% CI: 6.9 mmHg lower to 2.3 units higher), $p = 033$. Results suggest a tendency to lower levels of blood pressure if pregnant women, waiting for their clinic appointments, do so in the presence of live music.

d. The effect of live music on mothers and their unborn children

Preliminary results indicate that the heartbeat of the unborn child or foetus responds to music in a way that is medically consistent with fetal well-being. Full results of this study will soon be published, and we hope that the scientific evidence of these beneficial effects for mother and unborn child will lead to the introduction of live music in antenatal care programmes, thus enhancing the value of maternity services.

Conclusion

The philosophy behind Chelsea and Westminster Hospital Arts' activities has always been to be bold, to challenge expectations, and to bring the best of contemporary art and multicultural live performance to everyone, as part of the daily routine of the hospital. This ambitious and pioneering programme means that Chelsea and Westminster Hospital was the ideal place for asking how and why an arts programme can work in health care. The second and third phases of our research explore the feasibility –

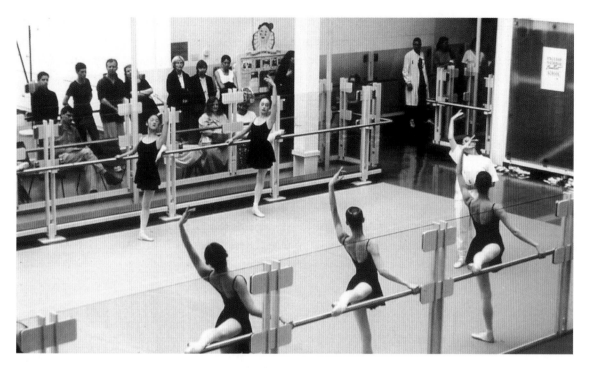

questioned by many – of measuring physiological and biological changes in patients receiving treatment in the presence of visual or performing arts, and in their absence. Preliminary results are very promising and further studies are under way.

Research studies have, for instance, shown that physiological and psychological stress result in increased blood pressure, high levels of circulating stress hormones – such as cortisol – and decreased immune responses.[15] Our current research therefore aims to assess whether the arts can help provide an environment conducive to diminishing levels of stress and anxiety[16] as reflected in these physiological markers. The level of cortisol and the amount of induction agents before anaesthesia will be measured in the day surgery unit, and in an orthopaedic ward; in addition the length of hospital stay, and the amount of analgesics consumed by patients recovering from the same type of operation, will be measured in the presence of the visual arts – including paintings on the ceilings of anaesthetic rooms – and live music. Controls will experience the same clinical care, in the same setting, and with the same staff, but will not be exposed to either works of art or live music.

A demonstration that the arts can change outcomes of clinical significance is vital if the burgeoning arts in health movement is to

Students at the neighbouring English National Ballet School are among the numerous music, drama, dance and art students who are given the opportunity of broadening their horizons by working at the hospital.

persuade hospital managers and clinicians to rethink their health care provision. The results suggest that our research will provide clear evidence of the kind required, and that there is indeed much to be gained in terms of patient satisfaction, staff morale, and improved patient outcomes from the integration of the arts in health care. We hope that the knowledge and experience we have gained will be of value to all who are interested in innovation and change.

Acknowledgements

The first year of this research was funded by the Research Committee of Chelsea and Westminster Healthcare NHS Trust Charity. The last two years of the project were funded by the King's Fund.

References

1 Behrman P. Art in hospitals: why is it there and what is it for? *The Lancet* 1997;**350**:584–5.

2 National Art Collections Fund Prize Programme, 1996.

3 Scher P, Senior P. *The Exeter evaluation*. Exeter: Royal Devon and Exeter Hospital, 2000.

4 Zigmond AS, Snaith RP. The Hospital Anxiety and Depression Scale. *Acta Psychiatr Scand* 1983;**67**:361–70.

5 Zeki S. Artistic creativity and the brain. *Science* 2001;**293**:51–2.

6 Miles MFR. Art in hospitals: does it work? A survey of evaluation of arts projects in the NHS. *J R Soc Med* 1994;**87**:161–3.

7 Meyrick J, Sinkler P. *An evaluation resource for healthy living centres*. London: Health Education Authority, 1999.

8 Lawson B, Phiri M. Room for improvement. *Health Service J* 2000;**24**: 20–23.

9 Hallam S. *The power of music*. London: The Performing Right Society, 2001.

10 Olson SL. Bedside musical care: applications in pregnancy, childbirth, and neonatal care. *J Obstet Gynecol Neonatal Nurs* 1998;**27**:569–75.

11 Wilkinson J. *Music in healthcare project: evaluation report*. Dublin: Music Network, 2000.

12 Francis S, Glanville R. *Building a 2020 vision: future health care environments*. London: The Stationery Office, 2001.

13 Staricoff RL, Duncan J, Wright M, Loppert S, Scott J. A study of the effects of the visual and performing arts in healthcare. *Hospital Development* 2001;**32**:25–8.

14 Wyn Owen J, 'Art, health and well-being: why now? The policy advisor's view'. In: Kirklin D, Richardson R (eds). *Medical humanities: a practical introduction*. London: Royal College of Physicians, 2001.

15 Burns SJ, Harbuz M, Hucklebridge F, Bunt L. A pilot study into the therapeutic effects of music therapy at a cancer help center. *Alternative Therapies* 2001;**7**:48–56.

16 Ulrich R. How design impacts wellness. *Healthcare Forum J* 1992;**10**: 20–25.

6

The effect of colour and design in hydrotherapy: designing for care

JANE DUNCAN

Public artist Jane Duncan describes the transformation of a dull hydrotherapy unit by the installation of 'Kites', a colourful abstract design. The artwork was created with the very specific clinical uses of the setting, and the users of that space, in mind. While patients were relatively quick to recognise the new environment as an improvement, staff took longer to appreciate the change.

Seeing comes before words

– John Berger[1]

Introduction

This chapter outlines the design, implementation and evaluation of a project which used art to transform a hydrotherapy unit from a merely functional space to one designed to engage both patients and staff.

One of the most rewarding and certainly one of the most challenging sites of activity for a public artist is that of the health care environment. The practical demands of any busy clinical setting require the artist to engage in a creative process which goes beyond the physical site, transcends the institutional, and integrates the historical, social and cultural identities which interact with the medical. Given that the work of a public artist is site-specific rather than gallery-oriented, a clinical environment appropriately provides all of these opportunities.

> The primary definition of public art has become predomi-
> nantly concerned with the primacy of the artist producing

studio work for a public setting: the activity of taking art out of the gallery and into the public space.[2]

Because a hospital is a unique environment, quite different from any other site, 'appropriateness and suitability are crucial':[3] consideration must be given not only to the architectural environment, but equally to the response of users, namely patients, staff and visitors. In this context, public art can act as a pivotal tool, counterbalancing the sometimes unappealing consequences of an environment shaped by clinical need, by integrating appropriate colour and design.

Until recent years, unless they were art therapists or teachers working directly with patients, artists did not generally frequent hospitals. Fortunately the climate is now changing, and the last decade has seen the role of the arts in health care grow in profile both in the UK and abroad. My own interest in the potential role of the visual arts in health care environments began in my student days when I became increasingly curious about the impact that art had on the emotions of the viewer.

Most of the hospitals I was familiar with at that time had a sterile, clinical feel about them, with very little to raise the spirit: waiting areas strewn with pamphlets and magazines, and only the occasional token picture for distraction. I began to question why this was so.

Why, when people are sick, often at their lowest ebb in life, should they also be subjected to a non-supportive environment? Why should the quality of the environment not match the standards of medical care? Why are the walls usually white, and why typically is the only aesthetic distraction a pathetic plant in the corner of the room? One of the most widely quoted academic papers on this subject, Roger Ulrich's 'View through a window may influence recovery from surgery',[4]* prompted me to ask further questions.

In his paper, Ulrich discusses the clinical benefits and restorative effects of offering a room with a view of trees, rather than a view of a brick wall, to recover in after surgery. The question of whether the visual environment plays any significant role in

---

*Records on recovery after cholecystectomy of patients in a suburban Pennsylvania hospital between 1972 and 1981 were examined in this study to determine whether assignment to a room with a window view of a natural setting might have restorative influences.

recovery was clearly answered by the results from the study, which identified that patients recovering with a view had shorter post-operative stays and required fewer analgesics than those with the brick wall.

Although the paper answered a vital question, it raised many others. Was it possible that visual art and colour could also make a significant difference to patient well-being and recovery? Could these responses be scientifically measured, physiologically and psychologically?

I became increasingly convinced that colour and design could be powerful tools for creating a more supportive environment. An inspiring lecture on 'Music and the mind' given by Professor Paul Robertson of the Medici String Quartet and Visiting Professor of Music and Psychiatry at Kingston University, reinforced this view; if music could have such a powerful transformative effect on the human being, then was it possible to find evidence that visual art might also? At the lecture I met Dr Rosalia Staricoff, Director of Research Projects at Chelsea and Westminster Hospital Arts, and we exchanged thoughts about these ideas. Shortly after, I was invited by the Hospital Arts Director, Susan Loppert, to join Dr Staricoff as Research Assistant at Chelsea and Westminster.

Background

The application and use of colour is not a new phenomenon–colour has been influencing artists and intriguing scientists for hundreds of years. Certainly by the nineteenth century, artists working with colour theory had become increasingly interested in scientific treatises, particularly Isaac Newton's *Opticks* (1704), and the discovery of the colour spectrum in daylight.[5] Further aspects of colour theory most interesting to artists have been theories of colour harmony, such as Newton's systemised circular colour diagram,* and the question of how colours relate to mechanisms of perception and affect the feelings of the spectator.[6]

---

*Although colour diagrams had been around since the fifteenth century, Newton arranged complementary colours of the spectrum in a circle opposite each other. Complementaries are pairs of colours that cancel each other out when mixed, to produce white if they are coloured lights and grey if they are coloured paints.

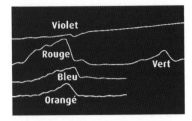

This graph originally appeared in a 1887 publication by French physiologist Charles Féré, *Sensation et mouvement*, and is reproduced in John Gage's book *Colour and culture*. Charles Féré measured the effect of exposure to different coloured lights on the contraction of muscles in the forearm of patients being treated for hysteria. As the graph demonstrates, the intensity of muscular contraction recorded was dependent on the wavelength, or colour, of the light to which the patient was exposed.

The development of colour theories, however, was not limited to scientists. The artist Kandinsky, in his 1912 essay 'On the spiritual in art',[7] introduced the concept of emotional values of colour as a language. Developing his theories directly from Goethe's *Theory of colours* (1810),[8] Kandinsky suggested that 'in general colour is a means of wielding a direct influence on the soul. Colour is the musical key. The eye is the hammer. The soul is the pianoforte with its many chords'.[7] Kandinsky was not alone in proposing that colour and form constituted a language of affects. According to the spiritual-philosophical beliefs of people like Rudolph Steiner and the philosopher Annie Besant, colours were interpreted, as they were experienced, in auras or 'thought forms'.[9]

Many of these early investigations into responses to colour also reinforced attitudes to synaesthesia – a condition associated with non-discrimination between the senses – and chromotherapy, the use of coloured light in healing. As John Gage notes in his book *Colour and meaning*, the early practical application of colour was related primarily to a question of feelings rather than of intellectual judgement.[6] However, what is less well evidenced but of increasing interest today is the influence and supporting evidence of the effect of colour, physiologically and psychologically.

Early scientific investigation into the physiological effect of colour is recorded in the late nineteenth century by Charles Féré, who first tabulated the effect of colour on muscular action on humans in 1887.[10] An interest in the phenomenon of colour has continued throughout the twentieth century, and the use of colour for health, architecture and commercial purposes is gaining increasing momentum. As cultures diversify, interest in the subject of colour is deepening and its applications becoming broader. Colour is more than simply a design tool: it contains values in its own right.[6]

One of the earliest examples of the practical implementation of colour for health and safety was at the outbreak of World War II. Millions of inexperienced men and women entered industrial jobs; as a result the accident rate rose rapidly. Faber Birren, an artist by training, devised a colour-coding system in an attempt to lower the accident rate. Accidents fell sharply after his system was introduced. The US Navy also recorded a 28% decrease in their accident rate after taking up his recommendations.[11] Birren's colour safety codes became internationally recognised, and his specifications are still applied in industrial and commercial buildings today.

Almost half a century later, in an article published in 1984, PK Kaiser reviewed the literature on the non-visual physiological effects of colour on humans. He emphasised how different studies have shown that colour can influence electrical patterns of the brain, galvanic skin response, blood pressure, heart rate, respiration rate, eye blink frequency and blood oxygenation.[12] He concluded that 'there are reliably recorded physiological responses to colour in addition to those generally associated with vision.'[13] Further research into physiological responses to colour, and the question of whether red is a more activating colour than blue, is discussed in a paper by Byron Mikellides, 'Colour and physiological arousal'. His paper addresses 'two schools of opposing thought':

> One is based on coloured light and measured by physiological changes in the central and autonomic nervous system and the other based on coloured pigment applied in interior and exterior spaces while varying the dimensions of hue, chromatic strength, and lightness of the colours. An experiment is discussed where subjects experience realistic full scale red and blue spaces and where both physiological and affective measures are taken ... This paper concludes in support of previous research in the field, that chromatic strength (saturation of a colour) is the key to affecting how exciting or calming a colour is perceived to be, and not the dimension of hue as previously thought by colour design manuals.[14]

These studies encourage the belief that colour has more than an aesthetic role to play in the successful design of our environment, but there remain many unanswered questions.

At the University of Leeds, Dr Jim Nobbs, Director of the Colour Chemistry Department, is beginning to uncover some of the complexities surrounding our emotional responses to colour. In collaboration with the Kyoto Institute of Technology in Japan, and other international groups, he has devised a set of colour emotional scales to scientifically evaluate emotional responses to colour.

The Nobbs' Scales are based on word pair analysis: a single colour sample relating to the PANTONE MATCHING SYSTEM®, an international printing, publishing and packaging colour language, is

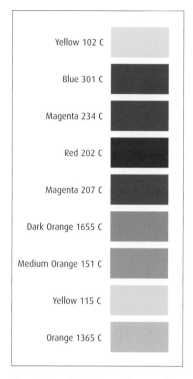

Figure 1 The nine Pantone colours used in the Nobbs word pair analyses.

The PANTONE MATCHING SYSTEM is an international printing, publishing and packaging colour language providing an accurate method for the selection, presentation, specification, communication, matching and control of colour. PANTONE® and other Pantone, Inc. trademarks are the property of Pantone, Inc.

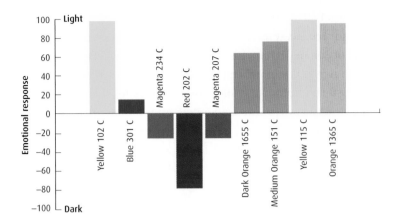

Figure 2 Nobbs' colour emotional scale for the word pair 'Light/Dark'

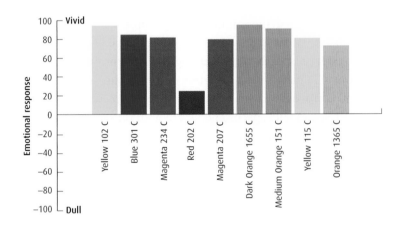

Figure 3 Nobbs' colour emotional scale for the word pair 'Vivid/Dull'

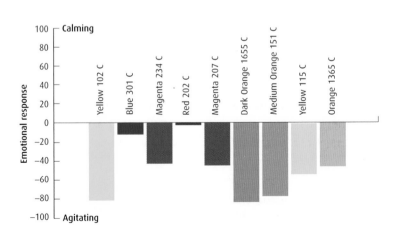

Figure 4 Nobbs' colour emotional scale for the word pair 'Calming/Agitating'

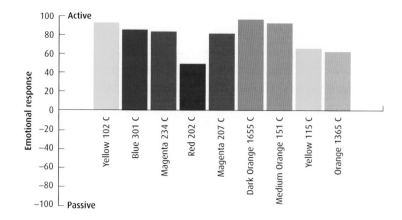

Figure 5 Nobbs' colour emotional scale for the word pair 'Active/Passive'

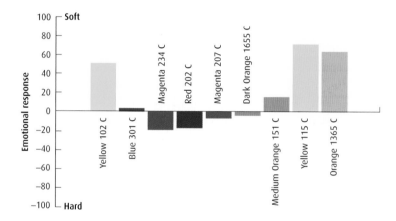

Figure 6 Nobbs' colour emotional scale for the word pair 'Soft/Hard'

given to the viewer together with a word pair opposite, eg dark/light. The viewer responds by scoring the colour on a sliding scale.

'Bright', 'strong', 'vivid', 'warm', are words that people might use to describe their impression of the colour of a surface. Some of the words may be chosen with the intention of conveying the visual attributes of the appearance, the hue, the lightness and the intensity of the colour, and other words chosen are an attempt to convey an 'emotional' response that the observer associates with the colour's appearance. The technique of analysis involves listing pairs of colour descriptive antonyms, such as 'Active/Passive'. Under controlled conditions, the observers are passed a variety of coloured panels from which they select words from a list which they believe best describe their impression of the coloured panel. The judgements are repeated with a series of coloured panels and then analysed scientifically using the Nobbs scientific formula.

Although the development of colour scales has been treated with scepticism by the established community of colour physicists, they are of considerable interest to people involved in selecting colours on the basis of these very properties. Examples include designers working with graphics, packaging and textile materials, as well as interior designers and architects.[15]

The brief

Every public art commission is a blend of creative ideas and original concepts but what made this commission unique was the decision to incorporate it into the research project.

The hydrotherapy room was a cold, white clinical space, lit by fluorescent-strip lighting and a four-panelled frosted glass window, with the pool in the centre of the room. Other than a clock on the wall, assorted equipment and a selection of information sheets, there was no visual diversion or stimulus of any kind. The hydrotherapy unit was used by a variety of patients, from those with hip replacements to children with long-term neurological difficulties. Consequently a patient's requirement for sessions would vary considerably from one or two sessions a week to a session every few months, depending on the condition. Both staff and managers agreed that the unit could benefit from a visual transformation.

The brief was to design murals for the walls and ceiling of

The hydrotherapy room before the commission of 'Kites' (opposite and overleaf) was a cold, white, clinical space, lit by fluorescent-strip lighting and a four-panelled frosted glass window. Design considerations including camouflaging the fire bell, and drawing attention to the fire exit and emergency equipment.

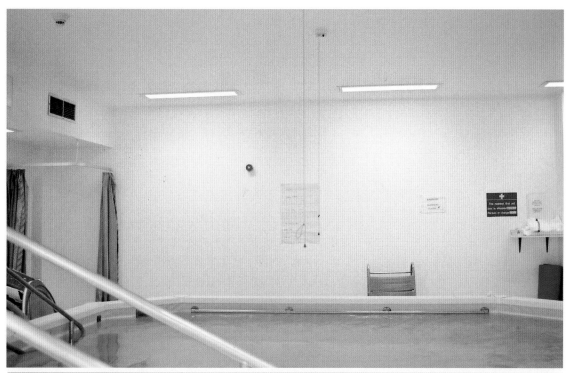

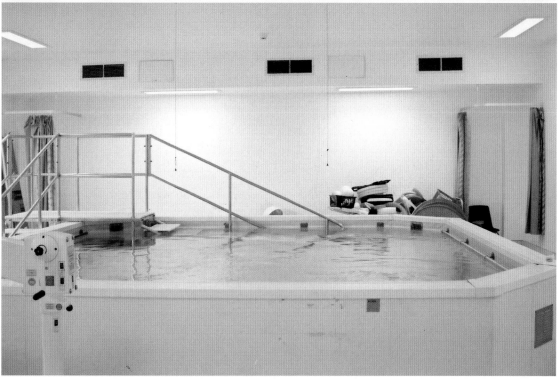

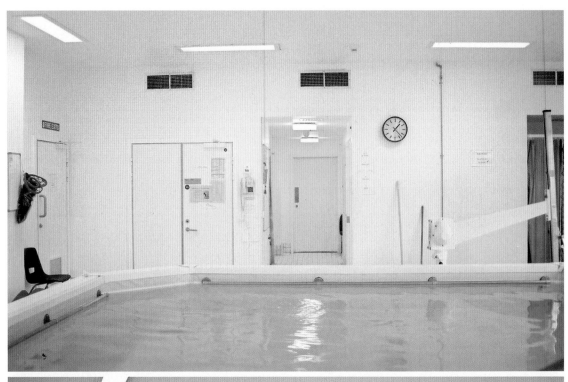

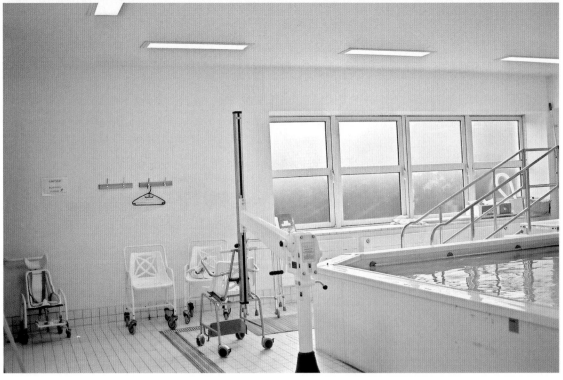

the hydrotherapy room, and to transform the clinical environment, using warm, bright colours and bold abstract design. The objective was to create an environment which would be stimulating for patients, a catalyst for physical movement, a visual aid for staff when treating patients, and a pleasurable environment to work in. As the hospital serves a wide cross-section of the multicultural community, it was considered important that the design did not inadvertently resemble any specific national flag, sign or symbol.

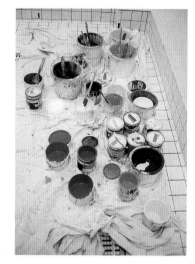

The colours of the paint were precisely mixed and applied in three layers in order to achieve exactly the right tone.

Preparation and safety issues

One of the most important aspects of any commission is the preparatory work. In a hospital this includes obtaining support and approval from every relevant quarter, as well as attending to health and safety requirements. Preparing well at the beginning of the commission helps free the mind to enjoy the creative process to come.

Every commission has unique circumstances which need to be considered. For this project they were the possible effects of lingering paint odour and the need to cover the pool area to provide safe access to the ceiling. Time was also a key limiting factor; just three days, over a weekend, were allowed to complete the entire project, and since patients would need to use the pool immediately after it was finished it was essential to use a paint without an odour that would permeate the atmosphere and cause discomfort and irritation to staff and patients.

Since the smell of oil paint can linger for days, it was rejected in favour of acrylic paint. Also, because of the time constraints, it was decided to cover the surface of the pool rather than to drain it. Plastic sheeting was spread across the pool, and scrupulous attention was given to sealing the edges to prevent any particles of dust entering the water. The ceiling was reached by a system of steel planks on trestle supports.

The design

Colour harmony must rest on a corresponding vibration in the human soul; and this is one of the guiding principles of our inner need.
  – Kandinsky[7]

It was a colourist's dream to be asked to design a mural for this stark white space, which lacked any sense of identity or energy. A set of designs and colours was carefully selected, using a palette of nine colours, each corresponding to the Pantone® colour system and later evaluated using the Nobbs Colour Emotional Scales (see Fig 1).

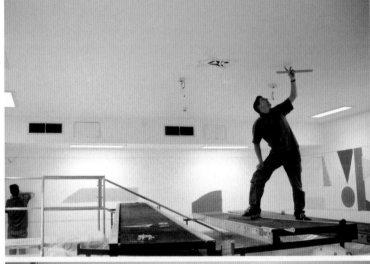

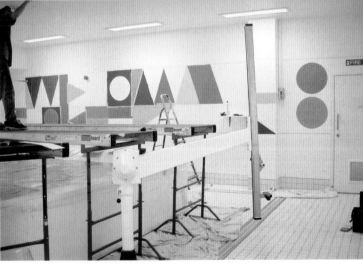

Above, steel tressel supports are used in order to access the ceiling. Below, the design begins to take shape; the first layer of colour is applied, and two bold orange circles in different tones clearly mark the fire exit. The fire bell can be seen, before its camouflage within the design, on the far wall to the left of the picture.

The designs incorporated bold colours and geometric shapes linked to form a continuous abstract pattern across the walls, with a complementary design on the ceiling. Lines and colours were carefully positioned, in order that they could be used as an aid by staff during treatment. Children with special needs are often supine in the water when they use the pool, so special attention was therefore given to the ceiling, the obvious focal point of the room. The emergency equipment and fire exits were highlighted by the use of specific colours and shapes, in contrast with other wall fixtures such as towel pegs, which were carefully camouflaged so that there was no interruption to the design. Working

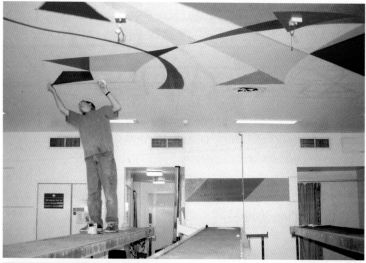

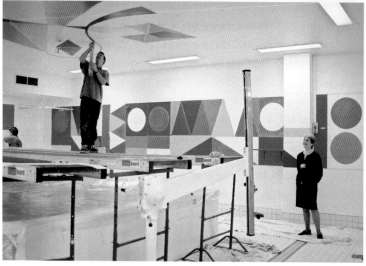

Above, mapping out the ceiling. Lines and colours are carefully measured and positioned, and the designs begin to transform the environment as each layer of colour is applied. An interested visitor watches the work (below).

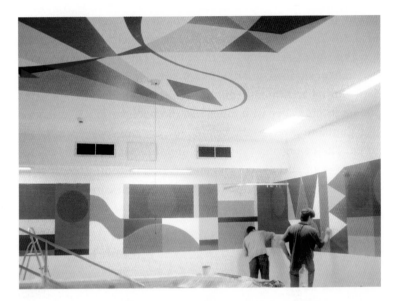

Precise painting created crisp lines and sharpened the design. The fire bell, now camouflaged, can just be made out within the red square on the right wall.

with paint on such a large scale, and with the added need to paint three layers of each colour in order create the right tone, the project required careful planning, particularly as there was so little time to complete the work. Due to the timescale the assistance of two other painters was necessary.*

In three days the hydrotherapy room was completed, transformed from a cold, stark clinical environment to a warm, vibrant and invigorating space. The mural is, appropriately, entitled 'Kites'.

Evaluation

After consultation with medical staff an existing questionnaire, already in use within the Chelsea and Westminster Research Project,[16] was modified for use in this study. The questionnaire was distributed in three phases: before the murals were painted, in the first month after the painting, and three months after.

The aim was to generate both quantitative and qualitative data from both patients and staff about their responses to the changes in the hydrotherapy room. In addition, this study afforded an opportunity to evaluate the effect of the colours used in the design. The system used to evaluate the effect of the colours was the Nobbs Colour Emotional Scales.

---

*Grateful thanks are due to Jonathan Brunson and Jason Burke.

Results

Overall approval ratings of staff and patients

There was no significant increase in the approval ratings of either patients or staff one month after the installation of 'Kites'. After three months, however, patients rated the changes to the environment significantly more positively than in the first month. Interestingly, after three months patients responded to the changes more positively than staff: 68% of patients considered the colours and designs improved the environment, compared to 29% prior to the installation.

There was no significant change in staff responses after three months. However, some of the staff reported they found the colours and designs were helpful, as they acted as a focal point when treating patients, particularly children.

One possible explanation for why responses were less positive at one month than at three months is the natural resistance we all

The design incorporated bold colours and geometric shapes linked to form a continuous abstract pattern across the walls, with a complementary design on the ceiling.

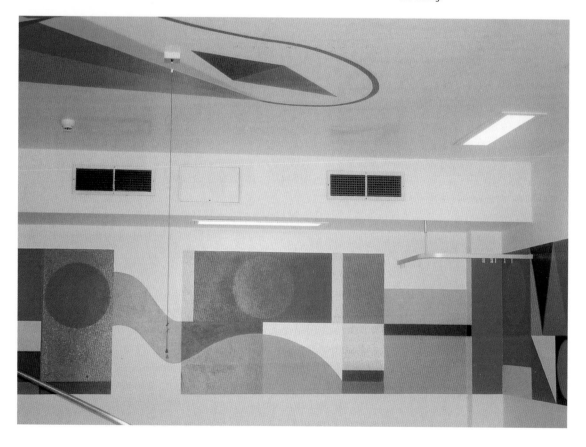

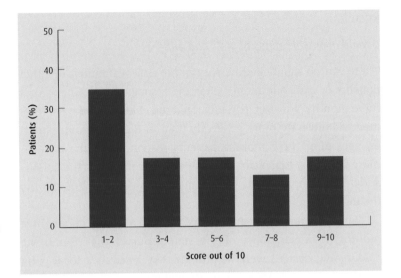

Figure 7 Patient responses, after one month, when asked to rate the change in the hydrotherapy unit on a scale of 1 to 10, where 1 equals for the worse and 10 equals for the better.

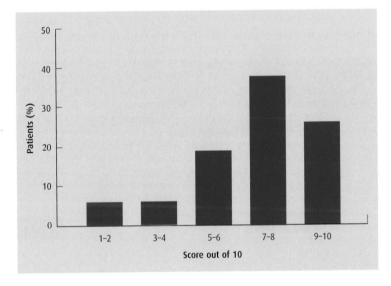

Figure 8 Patient responses, after three months, when asked to rate the change in the hydrotherapy unit on a scale of 1 to 10, where 1 equals for the worse and 10 equals for the better

have to change. In general people adapt poorly to change, and the hydrotherapy room went through a particularly dramatic transformation in only a few days. Despite the fact that staff were consulted beforehand it may have been somewhat disconcerting for them to leave a white room on Friday evening and return to a kaleidoscope of colour on Monday morning. Adapting to dramatic changes in our visual environment is perhaps a slower process than we might imagine, or even like to admit. It may take time for staff to accept a new identity in a space and develop a sense of ownership.

Responses to specific colours

How patients and staff would respond to specific colours was uncertain. Previous research has shown that certain colours are associated with action and movement[10] and these research findings influenced the choice of colours used in my design. The fact that patients would only spend short periods of time in the pool was also taken into account. Some of the results were surprising. One of the yellows, Pantone 102 C, which had an exceptionally high 'vivid' content, was also considered to be fairly 'soft' by respondents. Equally surprising was the fact that red Pantone 202 C, which is usually considered to be an active colour, scored lowest on the 'active/passive' scale, and neutral when evaluated as being 'soft' or 'hard', 'calming' or 'agitating'. Perhaps the most surprising result was from the blue Pantone 301 C, which was rated almost equally as 'vivid' as 'active', and unusually neutral when analysed as 'soft' or 'hard'. Even more curiously, it was high on the 'agitating' scale. The majority of the responses were, however, consistent with Nobbs' research findings.

Special attention was given to the ceiling, the obvious focal point of the room. Children with special needs are often supine in the water when using the pool.

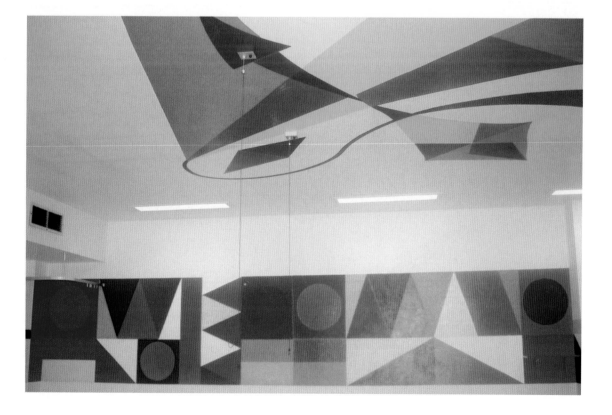

Conclusion

The results of this study suggest that artists must continue to ask probing questions about what is acceptable and valuable in the design of working environments. Nevertheless, the overwhelmingly positive response of users to the commission after three months provides reassuring justification for both the colour and design changes. Essentially, it reflects the need to progress ideas about how to address the design of hospitals and working environments of the future. There are many choices, and many questions remaining, such as how we can optimise the use of colour and art to help transform institutional and clinical environments in the most appropriate way. If specific colours and designs are successful in hydrotherapy, how can we define what are the most appropriate compositions and colours for other clinical settings? Which combination of colours and compositions works best? How can we measure which are the most appropriate colours and designs?

Ceiling detail. The mural is, appropriately, entitled 'Kites'.

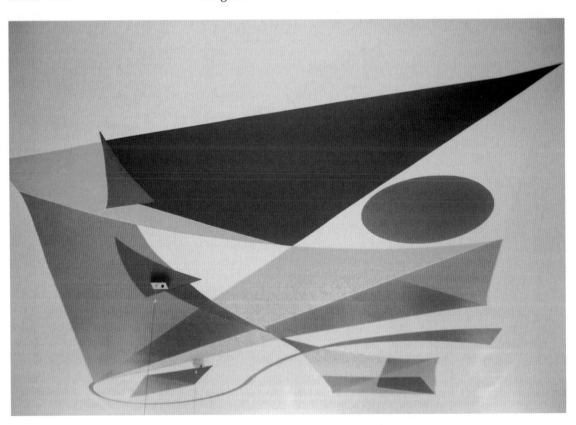

We live in an evidence-based society, and such research is vital to support the progression of ideas about how we continue to implement and accept changes to our visual environment. Encouragingly, the space in which patients receive hydrotherapy at the Chelsea and Westminster Hospital continues to be a lively focus of activity, and although this study clearly raises important questions, it has provided compelling evidence of the fundamental benefits of the use of appropriate colour and design in the health care environment. These benefits are more than just an improvement in aesthetic appeal. The application of appropriate colour and design in a clinical setting can not only enhance the experience of patients during treatment, but can also help create a positive sense of well-being for staff, providing a stimulating and supportive working environment.

References

1   Berger J. *Ways of seeing.* London: Penguin, 1990.

2   *Art and Architecture.* 2002, No 57.

3   Loppert S, '*Ars gratia sanitatis*: the art of the possible'. In: Haldane D, Loppert S (eds). *The arts in health care: learning from experience.* London: King's Fund, 1999.

4   Ulrich R. View through a window may influence recovery from surgery. *Science* 1984; 224:420–21.

5   Green J. *Pocket guides: colour.* London: The National Gallery, 2000.

6   Gage J. *Colour and meaning: art, science and symbolism.* London: Thames and Hudson, 1999.

7   Kandinsky W, 'On the spiritual in art' 1912. Quoted in: Mondadori A. *The history of art.* Milan, 1989.

8   Goethe JW, 'The theory of colours'. Quoted in: Gage J. *Colour and meaning. art, science and symbolism.* London: Thames and Hudson, 1999.

9   Besant A, 'Thought forms, Lucifer, a theosophical monthly'. Quoted in: Gage J. *Colour and meaning: art, science and symbolism.* London: Thames and Hudson, 1999.

10 Féré C, 'Sensation et mouvement'. Quoted in: Gage J. *Colour and meaning: art, science and symbolism.* London: Thames and Hudson, 1999.

11 Birren F. *Color psychology and color therapy.* New York: McGraw-Hill, 1950.

12 Kaiser PK. Physiological response to colour: a critical review. *Colour Research and Application* 1984:**9(1)**;29–35.

13 Brainard GC. 'The biological and therapeutic effects of light.' In: Nassau K (ed). *Colour for science, art and technology*. Amsterdam: Elsevier, 1998.

14 Mikellides B. Colour and physiological arousal. *J Architect Planning Res* 1990;**7**:1.

15 Nobbs J, 'Characterisation of emotional response to colour', presented at NPL Optical Radiation Measurement Club, 'Colour, Lighting and the Therapeutic Benefits', London, May 2002.

16 Staricoff RL, Duncan JP, Wright M, Loppert S, Scott J. A study of the effects of the visual and performing arts in health care. *Hospital Development* 2001;**32**:25–28.

7

The Mind Arts Project in Stockport: community arts in action

MICHAEL ANDERSON

Michael Anderson, manager of the Mind Arts Projects in Stockport, describes the first eight years of a community arts project which aims to support and empower local people with mental health problems. By providing opportunities for creative self-expression, this project has allowed users to grow in confidence and independence, and enabled them to play a more active role in community life.

Aut lux hic nata est aut capta hic libera regnat. (Light was either born here or, held captive, here reigns free.)

   – Inscription in Ravenna, among the mosaics

Introduction

In this chapter I will describe the first eight years of a community arts project in Stockport, the Mind Arts Project in Stockport (MAPS), which was established in 1995 to address unmet needs of local people with mental health problems. I will set the stage by describing a number of projects currently being undertaken by members of MAPS. I will then provide some background information about why the arts are thought to be useful in helping patients with mental health problems, and why it was felt that there was a need for such a community-based project in Stockport. As well as allowing members or participants in the project to tell their own stories, I will tell the practical story of how MAPS was taken from an idea to reality and what that entailed. These stories are offered as both encouragement and guidance to those wishing to develop similar community arts programmes. Although there is no single blueprint for establishing a viable project, I will attempt to identify the essential elements of the approach we have taken at MAPS.

Setting the stage

Really we don't make theatre, we use theatre to make magic. I would measure the success of a show according to whether the magic works. It can happen that you play out of tune, you can fall over, but the magic will work. It can also be pouring with rain, or perhaps because it's pouring with rain, it is particularly magical. But what happens is some kind of release of energy that is special. There's a heightened awareness, and there's a communication between audience and makers and performers that is unusual and it's something that is a lot bigger than everybody. When it all comes together – the images, the sound, the flow of energy, the weather and the sense of well-being afterwards, that you've made something very special – that's very rare … it's the change of consciousness, which is crucial, rather than the producing of the fine product. The product can be very fine but if it doesn't have a reasonably profound effect on the changing of consciousness, then it's a waste of time.

    – John Fox[1]

'Art in a box' (2003) Artists, schools and community groups from as far afield as Italy, France and Australia responded to the invitation to contribute small artworks to this enormous exhibition, which included 258 separate works, all small enough to be sent in the mail. The exhibition took place in the MAPS gallery, which was established in 2000. This process was initiated by works created by our members, which were then mailed out with an invitation to send us something in return. The work on display was diverse and original, seemingly inspired by the restrictions of size imposed by having to make something for a box measuring only a few inches on a side. The work has all been added to our onsite gallery, which may be accessed from our website at www.mindartsproject.co.uk

I am writing this chapter in March 2003. To give you an impression of how dynamic this project has become in recent years, I will mention just a few of the things we are doing at present. To begin with, a team of members, volunteers and staff are currently putting together an exhibition called 'Art in a box'. This is a mail art exhibition, to be held in the MAPS Gallery in April, which will have over 200 works of art on display. Small boxes containing artworks from as far afield as Europe and Australia have been flooding in over the past few months, in response to those created and mailed out by MAPS members. At the same time, another group of MAPS members is working with our programme coordinator, Jacqui Wood, to write *City of dreams*, a radio play commissioned by the BBC for airing on World Mental Health Day, 10 October 2003. Meanwhile, the 15 members and three volunteers involved in the MAPS Hypothetical Theatre Company are currently hard at work on their latest production, *Stellar stories*. Under Jacqui's inspirational direction, the company has performed on several occasions at the Royal Exchange Theatre in Manchester. The company

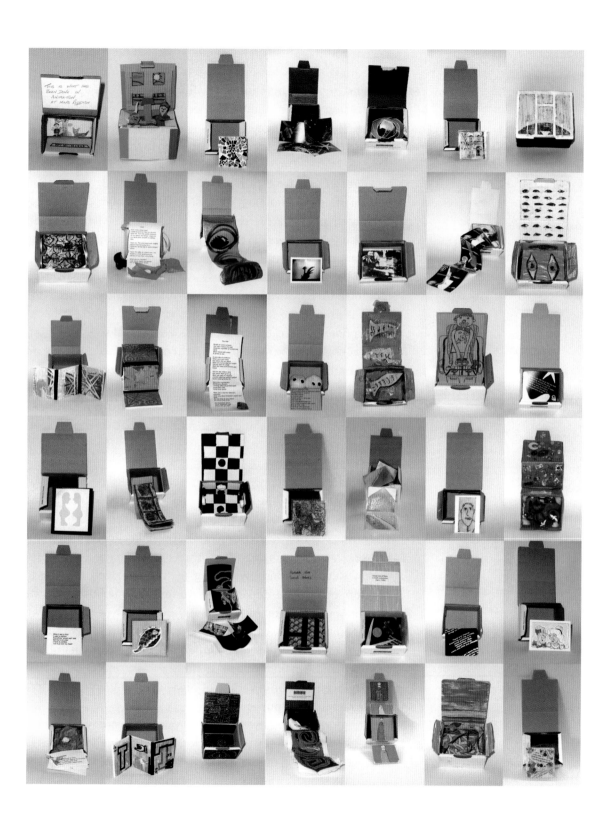

marched in the Streetworks Parade in May 2002. The theme for the parade was 'A feast of delights'. All of the costumes and banners (not to mention the dragon!) were designed and constructed by the members. The group then marched in the Jubilee Parade in Manchester in June of that year.

Film and animation projects completed in the past year include 'SPACED OUT!', 'Down to earth', and 'Dog in autumn time'. The creative writers have produced *Herd of words 2*, our second illustrated poetry anthology, published in December 2002. Large, laminated pages of *Herd of words 2* were assembled as an exhibition that toured several local libraries to coincide with the publication.

Our newsletter group is busy editing a glossy magazine to promote MAPS to a wider public. It is called *Insight*, and while the group is putting the finishing touches to it, media worker Sharon Tait is photographing all the mail art boxes for inclusion in our on-site gallery at **www.mindartsproject.co.uk**. *Insight* includes an article on the outreach work we have been doing on the psychiatric wards at Stepping Hill Hospital over the past five years, particularly a creative writing project which has had a measurable impact on the patients and ward staff. The magazine also spotlights two of our members who have made the difficult transition to art school recently.

A creative computing group has been established in the past few months and is rapidly increasing in membership. In the coming year some of our members will be trained in web design. They will soon be ready to take responsibility for updating our website. We are going to offer other organisations a service to design websites, which will bring in much needed revenue to develop our media department. Ultimately members will be providing this service, as they now produce our newsletter. Two photography groups continue to produce exciting, high quality imagery, and have contributed to the new website. Digital photography has been introduced in the past few months and has already been used in a variety of areas including animation, the newsletter and our publicity.

The mural group is working with our visual arts worker, Tess Hills, to produce mosaic commissions for Stepping Hill Hospital, the second major commission for the hospital in the past year. The group also produced a series of banners for com.art.02, the Greater

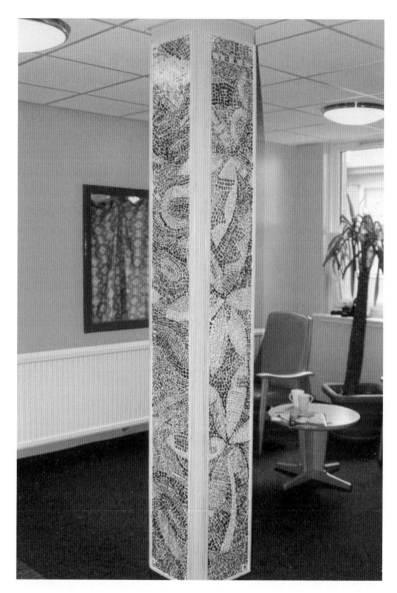

Mosaic pillar, Stepping Hill Hospital (2002) We are regularly commissioned to produce murals and mosaics for the local hospital. The two mosaic pillars for the Department of Psychiatry at Stepping Hill Hospital in 2002 involved over 20 members from our visual arts department. It has led to an offer of a further commission. In addition, we have been running outreach sessions on the wards since 1999, including art and writing sessions. We continue to develop this aspect of our work, as it enables us to reach those who are too ill to attend sessions in our Reddish Studios.

Manchester Community Arts Festival, which were displayed at the Zion Centre in Hulme, and several other commissions. In visual arts, more members than ever before are now purposefully developing their own work. At certain times the studio becomes a forest of easels. An astonishing range of work has been produced, including paintings, mosaics, banners, prints, textiles, and even a totem pole! In April, we will launch Friends of MAPS, coordinated by our administrator, Nola Smith, with which we aim to strengthen our ties to the local community. At the same time, *Insight* will be published. The website will be launched. 'Art in a box' will open to the public.

Much of the work described above is of high quality – and all of it is being produced by people suffering from serious mental illnesses, who have been stigmatised and socially excluded, whose self-esteem was at rock bottom before they joined us. Furthermore, only a minority of our hundred-strong membership would claim to have had any previous creative interest since leaving school. While some have always had a well established and abiding commitment to art in one form or another, most would say that they had had no clue that they might possess untapped creative potential before they joined us. Yet many are now producing stunning work.

On quite another level, members are becoming increasingly involved in running MAPS itself, participating in staff meetings, organising social events and outings, being trained to facilitate members meetings, and helping us to put in place strategies intended to make MAPS as inclusive and supportive as possible, particularly for the most vulnerable members, and the most recent inductees.

Why use the arts in mental health?

Connected problems require joined up solutions

   – 'Our healthier nation: a contract for health'[2]

An American study has shown that about a third of us will suffer mental illness in our lifetime and about one-fifth of us will suffer active mental illness in any year.[3] Projects such as MAPS help to rehabilitate people who have been hospitalised and are struggling to re-establish themselves in the community. As we are in constant contact with members of the project we can provide ongoing support, and we nurture and sustain links with other services as part of a coordinated approach to care.

Some research would suggest that a positive self-image is vital to an individual if she or he is to make the most of whatever lifestyle choices are available. For example, low self-esteem is often at the root of a range of negative thought patterns that mitigate against taking decisions in one's own self-interest.[4-6]

A person who feels little sense of control over their lives in general would be likely to feel little sense of control over their health and well-being.[7] Also, the development of coping skills has been shown to help individuals remain emotionally healthy in the face of adverse environmental stress.[8]

Why in Stockport?

The estimated levels of care for Stockport indicate that up to 91,350 people may experience significant levels of psychiatric morbidity, of which one-third will be recognised as having a mental disorder by a GP. This from a population of 290,000. A key health objective identified by Dr Stephen Watkins, the Director of Public Health for Stockport, is 'to minimise the social exclusion resulting from disability and dependence. This can be done by reducing the amount of disability and also by changing the way society excludes people with disability'.[9]

The MAPS ethos

In MAPS, the ethos must be described as 'survival of the weakest', inspired by the humanist outlook of members themselves. At MAPS, people have the opportunity to learn new skills and use them creatively. They produce work that often surprises by virtue of its technical expertise and imaginative content. Furthermore, they support and reinforce each other with constant praise. Creative expression is cathartic and potentially transformative. The recovery of one's sense of self is no less, in many cases, than a personal epiphany.

It is of strategic significance that MAPS is located in the voluntary sector. Stockport Health Authority's strategic framework for commissioning identifies a need for sustained partnership with the voluntary sector 'to enable people of all ages with mental illness to receive effective care and treatment in the most appropriate setting in accordance with needs'. 'The whole concept of Arts and Health is about nurturing an holistic attitude to healing and in improving the mental health of the community.'[9]

The proactive involvement of members in MAPS encourages them to feel that they are making a contribution to the project as a whole. They have control over their participation in creative activities and are active members of teams developing group work. They help to run the project itself. This addresses 'the need for social support ... affectionate relationships, the acceptance and significance given by others, membership of a group, respect, approval, self-respect and dignity, freedom and self-fulfilment... the need for participation and inclusion in society'.[10]

Largely inspired by their own efforts, members have made of MAPS a viable community, perhaps as tolerant, humane and inclusive as they would like society at large to be. 'So mental health is more like a journey than an arrival. But it is also deeply dependent upon the influences of society that make the journey either enjoyable, fulfilling, and worth doing, or arduous, despairing and without any sort of perceived worth or virtue'.[10]

MAPS is not unique. There are many mental health arts projects around the country. MAPS was established in 1995, but other projects have been around longer, such as the Start Studios in Manchester, Core Arts in London, and Trongate Studios in Glasgow. Some, like MAPS, are in the voluntary sector. Others are established within statutory services. Each project will have evolved according to local circumstances, though most will have in common a proactive membership and an inclusive approach to access. Like MAPS, most will have been established with the support of champions, individuals with influence and a pioneering spirit, who see a value in this type of work.

Getting MAPS up and running

A key person in the project's development was Peter Milnes, then Chief Executive of Stockport Health Authority. Crucial support also came from Adrienne Brown, Director of Stockport Arts and Health.

The idea of having a project of this kind in Stockport had first been proposed by Langley Brown, then Director of the Start Studios in Manchester. John Sculley, the Manager of Stockport Municipal Art Gallery, nurtured a small group of volunteers who were instrumental in getting the project off the ground. They were running a weekly art group at the gallery. The pilot work they did established the effectiveness of creativity in aiding recovery sufficiently to encourage them to think in terms of a full-scale arts project.

The group approached David Parker, Development Officer of the local Mind association, Stockport and District Association for

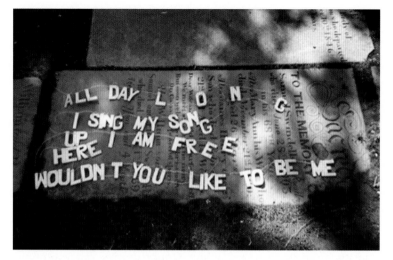

Chadkirk Sculpture Trail (1998) In 1998 we created a sculpture trail for Heritage Services at Chadkirk Chapel, a Romanesque building on the edge of ancient woodland. A variety of art forms were used in the creation of sculptures in wood, mosaic, straw and hessian. The centrepiece was a giant head, inspired by Easter Island and made of hessian stretched over a metal frame. Creative writing was transposed to 3D by making letters out of wood. Some of these poems were suspended between the trees, so they appeared to float above the woodland paths.

Mental Health, also known as Stockport Mind. Would they be willing to adopt the proposition for a full-time project? Stockport Mind had recently begun an expansion that continues to this day. They had already established counselling, befriending and outreach schemes, and were receptive to the idea of fostering and developing an arts project. A steering group consisting of the above stakeholders was established and funding obtained from two sources: The Consortium on Opportunities for Volunteering, a Department of Health funding scheme; and 'Joint Finance', a scheme for the creation of new projects jointly funded by Stockport Health Authority and Social Services. The funding from Opportunities for Volunteering was for three years only, that from Joint Finance tapered to the Health Authority over a period of seven years.

Sarah Berry, Development Officer for North West Mind, joined the steering group to monitor the expenditure of the Opportunities for Volunteering grant. I was appointed manager of the project in April 1995. I had a small operating budget and two rooms in Apsley Cottage, a small building in the centre of Stockport. Like my colleagues, I am a community artist. I came with a wide experience of community arts practice in England and abroad, including the USA, India, Bosnia and Slovenia.

I was actively seeking an opportunity to build a project from the ground up, having become frustrated with the peripatetic lifestyle of a freelance worker. In India and the USA, I had had direct experience of working in community centres where I could see the benefits of sustained development in establishing collective self-help, empowerment and social inclusion. One of my first tasks was to establish a referrals procedure and circulate information. Within three months the project had over 30 members. As membership built, I began to put in place a range of activities, including visual arts, creative writing, music and photography.

Since 1997, Stockport and District Association for Mental Health has had two divisions: Stockport Mind and MAPS. In 1995, though, MAPS was a small project managed by a sub-committee of the Association's management committee. The sub-committee developed out of the steering group that got the project started. The original intention was for MAPS to become an independent charity after three years, when Opportunities for Volunteers money ran out. In the event, MAPS and Mind decided to stick together, and MAPS became a co-equal division within the association. Together, we provide an exceptionally broad range of services. The vision of our management committee has been a key factor in the growth of the association. A succession of strong chairs and officers of committee have understood the value of a robust voluntary mental health sector in Stockport, participating in the delivery of services – sometimes to fill gaps in existing statutory services. The MAPS connection runs strongly throughout the Association: several former members, now volunteers, currently serve on our management committee and have a direct involvement in both divisions.

Blueprint for getting a community arts project started

▷ Identify the need for a project, adapted for local conditions
▷ Find a champion
▷ Set up a pilot project and gather evidence
▷ Create a steering group drawn from the arts, statutory and voluntary agencies, and service users
▷ Apply for funding from a range of sources
▷ Find appropriate facilities, preferably out in the community
▷ Appoint staff who believe in what they are doing

Richard's story

When I first went to MAPS, I was in a hostel for the homeless. I was unbelievably unhappy there. I had completely alienated my family. I guess MAPS became my family and without that support, there is every possibility that I wouldn't be around today. As a member, it offered me the chance to use creativity that I didn't know I had. I think the fact that Michael put so much faith in me, and was willing to let me become a volunteer, gave me responsibility, I mean that just brought my self-esteem and self-confidence flooding back. I can never put any sort of measurement on that, I don't know what would have happened if that hadn't been there for me.

– Richard Wickison, in an interview for *Insight* magazine

Richard Wickison is the present manager of Stockport Mind. It has flourished under his stewardship. The services it provides include counselling, advocacy, befriending, outreach, information services and a helpline. It has also fostered the development of 'Stuff' (Stockport User-Friendly Forum), a voice for change to improve mental health services, run entirely by service users.

Back in 1995, though, Richard was a service user himself. During his recovery from clinical depression, he started attending the weekly art group at Stockport Art Gallery, where I first met him on the day I was interviewed for the MAPS post. His is a remarkable story. Quite by chance, he became the very first member of MAPS. He worked closely with me in the early stages, when I was facing many challenges to the open-ended way in which I wanted the project to develop. He saw that my first concern was for the members. He also understood that I was determined to let MAPS evolve its own character, rather than duplicate existing models.

Within a few months he had become a volunteer with the project. In January 1996 he applied for the post of Stockport Mind's first advocacy worker. He established a highly respected and successful advocacy service, which is still going strong today. He was responsible for a successful lottery bid to purchase a larger building for Stockport Mind. For a brief time, he chaired the MAPS sub-committee, before eventually moving on to become manager of Tameside and Glossop Mind, where he remained for the next three and a half years. Tameside and Glossop Mind grew significantly under his management. A couple of years ago he returned to Stockport Mind, where he is applying the same successful formula for growth and development, strongly centred on the involvement of service users and partnership working with statutory services. The brief history of MAPS is full of such remarkable stories.

Membership

I was a real mess before I came here; I used to self-cut and tried suicide a couple of times. I'd be dead without MAPS. I'm here four days a week, otherwise I'd have no structure in my life.

  – A MAPS member, quoted in an external evaluation of MAPS

We receive referrals from a wide range of sources including community mental health teams, psychiatrists, therapists, psychologists, general practitioners and voluntary sector workers such as counsellors and advocates. Self-referrals are welcomed. At the referral stage, the emphasis is placed upon direct contact with the referrer, rather than on using a referral form. We work to build repeat custom and to develop an understanding of our culture among prospective referrers. A referral form is only used if the need for a risk assessment emerges in the conversation. That is, when there is a doubt regarding our capacity to include an individual who may be too ill, or too vulnerable.

We ensure that comprehensive information about the project is widely circulated, so that anyone who might benefit from attending may do so. The majority of referrers are comfortable sharing confidential information at this stage, understanding that this is essential to the process. (I know one social worker who prefers not to disclose such information until after the referred person has had a chance to visit the project, and the process has been adapted to allow for this.) On rare occasions when a referral is inappropriate, for example when an individual is outside our age range, we will do our best to ensure that they are referred on to a more appropriate agency such as Age Concern.

Once referred, a prospective member is invited to visit the project for a guided tour and a friendly chat. We make it clear at this stage that it is MAPS that is being assessed, not the visitor. The process is structured so that we may be confident of being able to offer a place by the time of the visit. The referrals process is under constant review. In October 2000 we introduced induction courses as a means of providing better support to new members. Each inductee receives a clear and comprehensive information pack, is given a taste of many of our activities, and is then encouraged to choose the groups they would like to join. This method has seen a significant reduction in the number of new members dropping out.

In April 2003, we will introduce a 'buddy' system, whereby experienced members will mentor new members in the early stages of their involvement. (The proposal for this innovation came from members themselves.) Each member's involvement is intensively supported and sustained. Links with referrers are maintained to ensure a coordinated response to each person's needs. Members are encouraged to let staff know when support is needed. Informal support is offered at all times. When a member encounters difficulties, help is provided. Members' well-being, involvement and personal development are our highest priorities.

Each member is reviewed regularly, to ensure that they are happy with the service, that they are receiving the support they need, and that they are being assisted in exploring other opportunities in education, volunteering and employment. Members have the option not to be reviewed if they prefer.

We have established a network of next step organisations including colleges, volunteer agencies and a sheltered employment agency. A member who wishes to explore other opportunities is supported through the process and encouraged to retain their membership as a safety net for as long as needed, even after they have stopped attending. For example, we know that ex-members find it comforting to remain on our mailing list. There is no time limit on membership, though we try to encourage each member to become progressively more independent.

Every year, the membership elects four representatives, two men and two women. These 'members reps' attend staff meetings and management committee meetings. They receive training to enable them to facilitate members' meetings, which take place every two months. A buffet is held after each members' meeting to establish a convivial atmosphere. Attendance at these meetings improved rapidly when these buffets were introduced.

The MAPS newsletter has already been mentioned. Produced almost entirely by members themselves, it allows them to publish their news, poems, stories, articles, photographs and illustrations.

Everyone can contribute. It is also, we have learned, an essential lifeline for members who are not attending, for whatever reason. As part of a quality assurance drive in 2000/2001, we established the practice of writing a year plan. Members participate in the planning process.

Increasingly, members are representing MAPS on the networking front. In 1997, two members travelled to Sheffield on behalf of MAPS to receive a Northwest Mind Positive Images award as part of National Mind's Respect campaign. Members have represented MAPS on various panels, including the Education Link group at Stockport College, the stigma and discrimination group and the World Mental Health Day consortium. They have also represented MAPS as delegates at the World Symposium of Arts and Health and the National Arts and Mental Health Forum. In the past year, four members have made the transition to volunteering within the project, with great success. Nevertheless, members' involvement in helping to run the project has plenty of scope for development, and the year plan for 2003/2004 will address this.

Blueprint for recruiting and supporting members

▷ Establish a referrals procedure and circulate information about the service

▷ Cultivate repeat custom to develop a network of referring agencies

▷ Pay close attention to the induction of new members

▷ Establish members' meetings and buffets

▷ Involve members in the planning process

▷ Encourage members to publish a newsletter to keep everyone in touch

▷ Involve members in networking

▷ Establish effective procedures for monitoring and evaluation

▷ Write a year plan

Taking off

In 1997 MAPS moved to larger and more suitable premises. As the manager of the project, I had realised that further growth in response to the demands of an expanding, empowered member-ship required more staff. As a consequence I wrote a business plan, and became a fundraiser.

The appointment of Jacqui Wood as part-time programme co-ordinator in 1997 was the outcome of this strategy. Jacqui came to us originally as a freelance arts worker in 1996, with a broad range of experience as a community drama worker, including two years as Youth Theatre Director at Contact Theatre in Manchester. She spent 1993 travelling and working abroad with youth and theatre companies in New Zealand, Australia and Canada, undertaking research and residencies sponsored by the British Council. She was drama animateur for Trafford Council from 1994 to 1999, when a successful bid for National Lottery Funding enabled us to make her post full time.

Jacqui's impact on programme development was instantaneous. She established drama and animation groups and, with her encouragement, members quickly grew in confidence. Teamwork began to flourish, leading to a more cohesive dynamic. An outreach strategy developed. In partnership with Heritage Services in 1998, MAPS members created a sculpture trail at Chadkirk Chapel with artist Noah Rose. In 1999, there was a unique exhibi-tion of MAPS work at Stockport Municipal Art Gallery, in which paintings, installations and gigantes were linked by poems pasted, graffiti-like, directly onto the walls. The drama group performed at the Royal Exchange Theatre in Manchester as part of com.art. The Hypothetical Theatre Company was established and marched in the Streets Ahead Parades in Stockport and Manchester.

The following year, we expanded further, taking on a large first floor unit. The MAPS Gallery was housed here, alongside rehearsal space for the theatre company, an animation studio, and later, a media department. More fundraising led to the creation of two new posts in 2001, for a visual arts worker and a media worker. Tess Hills, our visual arts worker, came to us from Australia, where she had been working in a community arts centre for several years. Media worker Sharon Tait is a college lecturer, who has also worked in settings similar to MAPS.

We began to earn income through a variety of commissions, to supplement our fundraising strategy. We added creative computing and digital photography to an already diverse pro-gramme. Through our own exhibition programme, publications, and 'Friends of MAPS', we have now begun to reach out to the community around us. By 2002, the project had over 100 members.

Heather Tease, a user of the MAPS project writes:

MAPS has proven to be a life-changing experience (with apologies for the cliché!). For (too) many years, I allowed 'work' to dominate my life. My self-esteem became totally wrapped up with 'the career'. I did not take care of myself. This led to the breakdown of my physical health and, career over, subsequent isolation, fear and depression.

It was scary at first to come to MAPS! In retrospect, the initial process was well structured, ie tour and then induction. However, for quite a while, it was scary to come to the sessions. Seeing the amazing pieces of art around, people working with a sense of purpose, seemingly already bonded, not really knowing anyone else. Daunting!

However, after this initial phase, I loved coming to MAPS. I felt a sense of MAPS being a safe place, which accepted me, as I was, where I was at, yet also able to engage me in the sessions. I now recognise this as the process whereby I developed that sense of acceptance of myself for myself, leading to growing confidence, which naturally spilled over into life outside MAPS. Hence, rather than feeling powerless, which produced a need to control, I am now in a place where I can simply be 'aware' and be accepting of the ebbs and flows of life, knowing all things will pass. Being free, I am no longer powerless or constrained by perceived threats and, equally, am open to new experiences.

I feel engaged not only in my own sense of well-being, but also that of MAPS.

MAPS provides a steadfast platform for me to explore my creative potential.

I am so proud to be a member of the MAPS community, which translates to:

Laughter   Fun   Sharing   Giving   Receiving   Caring
Encouraging   Challenging   Empathy   Possibilities

Turning to the recent past, the BBC project has taken my involvement in MAPS to a new level. I am thrilled to be part of the team, enjoying the creative process and bonding with my fellow writers. I am conscious of the values of commitment, loyalty and dedication as we support and encourage each other. Such a good feeling! A delight it will be when the play is aired. My pleasure is in the journey and also in knowing this will be yet another way to promote MAPS!

Working in strategic partnerships with statutory providers

We began to run sessions in statutory settings in 1998, such as mental health resource centres and psychiatric wards. Acting on our own initiative, we raised the funding to do this, having identified a gap in services for the most vulnerable clients; those trapped in their own homes, for example. To address this need, we established viable partnerships with community mental health teams and occupational therapists. In concert with them we developed a strategy of working in very small groups with support workers in attendance.

We have been running sessions in the Department of Psychiatry at Stepping Hill Hospital since 1999. Jacqui Wood, who oversees this work, explains:

I introduced creative writing to wards P3 and P4 in January 2002. Art sessions had been running on the psychiatric wards as part of the MAPS outreach programme for three years and I wished to build on the success of this work.

The writing sessions themselves began tentatively: the venue, by its nature, can be busy, unpredictable and distracting. I had to find a way to introduce a very personal, brave, and most importantly, unknown activity into this space. It seemed at first that patients and staff found it hard to see what we were doing – what creative writing really is. It's unlike painting or drawing, where work is immediately visible. So a selection of pieces written by patients was typed up, enlarged and laminated, and then displayed as an advert for the activity.

There have been times, with a really active group of patients on the wards, when I've arrived to find poems scribbled on scraps of paper and sellotaped over the top of and

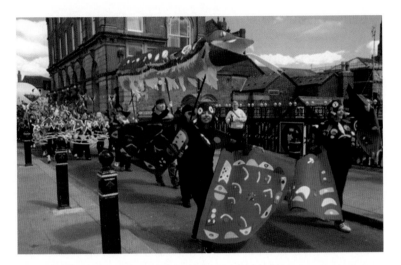

Streetworks Parade (2001) Our involvement in the Streets Ahead and later Streetworks parades in Stockport and Manchester began in 1999, preceding the establishment of the Hypothetical Theatre Company by Jacqui Wood in 2000. The company has been involved in numerous productions, performing at the Royal Exchange Theatre in Manchester on two occasions as part of com.art, the Greater Manchester Community Arts Festival.

around the laminated pieces – the poems spreading, creeping along the walls on both wards, and filling every available space. Like an infection.

Words on the wards challenge the assumption that seriously ill people are capable of nothing. This resistance, almost perversely, increases the impact of their success. The poetry-plastered walls are a testament to the intelligence and ability of the participants, all of them now writers.

– Jacqui Wood, 'The writing's on the wall'[11]

Volunteers

The role of volunteers has become more significant as the project has expanded. At any given time, anything from 15 to 20 volunteers will be involved, helping to run sessions, assisting our administrator in the office, and running our woodwork department. As our volunteers began to gain experience, we developed roles for them as freelance arts workers. To fill the gaps in our volunteering roster, we began to encourage members to make the transition to volunteering.

Pippa Kenyon, a volunteer who lives in the local community, explains why she chooses to work with MAPS:

I thoroughly enjoy working with everyone at MAPS. The project is fascinating, and it is wonderful to see how everyone benefits from time in the studio. All staff work extremely hard to bring a wide range of opportunities to members. Every day is different; although I work mainly on an administrative basis, which is my background, I have also been involved in various interesting arts projects and initiatives. I was welcomed into MAPS from the start, and feel as valuable as a permanent member of staff.

Does it work?

Monitoring and evaluation of outcomes is integral to our work process, and we routinely record the number of referrals made, the numbers that go on to take up a place after induction, the frequency of attendance, the numbers attending each studio session and the outcomes of membership. A recent questionnaire provided the following information about our members. In 2002/2003 MAPS had a total of 133 members, of whom 98 were current and 35 had left.

Of the 98 current members 40 were in need of support, six wanted to be a members' representative, nine to help with refurbishments, 17 to help with exhibitions, six to help run a session, nine to mentor other members and 25 wished to work as a volunteer at MAPS. Seventeen currently attend college, five volunteer elsewhere, and eight are in employment or with Worklink. Fourteen expressed an interest in attending college, 10 wished to volunteer elsewhere, eight were interested in becoming employed, and 12 wanted to increase their involvement in MAPS.

Of the 35 members who had left MAPS, five had moved into employment, four had started college education courses, six were working as volunteers and one had been referred on to other services. Eleven had relapsed, seven had left for other reasons and one had died.

As well as our own, internal evaluations, we feel that external and independent evaluation is helpful. We are a broad church, basing our work practice on the creative arts, across a wide range of specialisms. We have a great deal of experience and expertise within our field, have many skills and, contrary to popular misconception, are highly organised. Despite the fact that fully 65% of our annual budget is raised from non-statutory sources, and that our strategic value in a coordinated approach to needs depends on the independence this gives, we are nevertheless aware of the need to explain our work in terms funders and health professionals can measure. In

1999 we therefore commissioned an external evaluation of MAPS by an independent agency, Stockport Centre for Health Promotion.

The evaluation was conducted by Sarah Clarke between July 1999 and February 2000. The process involved extensive direct observation, numerous interviews, questionnaires, and data analysis. Everyone connected with the project was involved, including referrers. The final report was widely distributed within Stockport Health and Social Services, and copies were sent to various national agencies. This extract from the executive summary outlines the evaluating report's conclusions:

> This evaluation has observed and recorded the high degree of satisfaction and benefit that members experience as a result of participating in the project.
>
> It is an example to other projects and services of the high standards of creative achievement that can result from engaging people with limited knowledge and creative skills with artists in a dynamic project, which has a vision for individual and collective achievement.
>
> MAPS provides emotional, social and practical support enabling people with severe mental illness to stay within their own homes and the wider community. It provides a structure and a community for people to build their lives around, and the reduction in social isolation is considerable.
>
> The pride and sense of ownership members feel in the project is communicated by the members to mental health specialists in Stockport.
>
> A significant number move on to college or become volunteers outside the project. A small number move directly into work.
>
> MAPS is a multi-faceted project that operates at many levels. It balances vulnerable individuals' needs for support, creativity and social opportunity, the desire for sanctuary and safety from a hard external environment with the need of the project as a whole to continue to develop creatively and not become a stagnant institution.
>
> MAPS provides excellent value for money in the good quality of service it offers people with a high level of need.
>
> Further development of the project should be a key component in Stockport's mental health strategy as it plays

a key role in fulfilling the standards for mental health required by the government's National Service Framework, particularly Standard 1 and Standard 4.[12]

Blueprint for keeping going and keeping growing

▷ Locate suitable premises, which are spacious and airy
▷ Write a business plan
▷ Develop a fundraising strategy
▷ Establish and develop a rich and diverse programme
▷ Involve and train volunteers
▷ Create partnerships with other agencies
▷ Expand the staff team
▷ Raise the profile through exhibitions, performances and publications
▷ Develop outreach activities to meet gaps in services
▷ Commission an external evaluation

Conclusion

EURIPIDES: What do you want a poet for?
DIONYSUS: To save the city of course.

– Aristophanes, *The frogs*

At the heart of what we do rests the abiding conviction that creativity is innate and universal, and once permitted, has enormous power to transform us. It is like winning the lottery, except that everybody wins. It is profoundly moving to witness each member's journey to returning confidence and self-esteem. It is always such a personal thing.

We may also reflect upon the way in which their creative achievements – both singular and collective – utterly transform their image of themselves, and challenge us to reflect upon our common assumptions about mentality. Can we not be happy and ill at the same time? If so, then how is the relationship between mental health and mental illness to be understood? Causing us to question our assumptions is a consequence of the creative experience for all of us and this experience must be authentic, must be real, or it is not truly creative.

When we speak of social inclusion we are not merely spouting rhetoric, nor are we speaking of conformity. Members of MAPS are not necessarily interested in being like everybody else. They wish to be themselves, and to be accepted, even admired, for who they are. Why should they not take pride in strutting their stuff when they exhibit or perform?

Funding for organisations like MAPS is hard to obtain because of the negative image associated with mental illness. It is not a popular cause. Yet mental illness and mental health are not opposites that divide us. We simply have difficulty accepting that what our neighbour suffers is part of our shared condition. There is a saying from Africa; 'It takes an entire village to make one healthy child'.

In our society, fragmented as it is, the social component to mental illness is still to be universally accepted and understood. Yet almost half of those suffering from mental illness live alone.[9] Strangely, the only thing I know of that people fear more than mental illness is their unleashed creativity. Perhaps that is why taking the dare is so often the indicator of a return to health.

Creativity is more than just a bandage for the wound. What we create defines us. It enables us to recognise ourselves in what we create, and by this means to recognise each other. To be able to say, like the Roman orator Terence, 'Nothing human is alien to me'.

References

1 Quoted in: Coult T, Kershaw B. *Engineers of the imagination*. London: Methuen, 1983.

2 *Our healthier nation: a contract for health (Green Paper)*. London: The Stationery Office, 1998.

3 Robins L, Regier D. *Psychiatric disorders in America: the epidemiological catchment area study*. New York: Free Press, 1991.

4 Beck AT. *Cognitive therapy and emotional disorders*. Madison, CT: International Universities Press, 1976.

5 McKay M, Fanning P. *Self-esteem*. Oakland, CA: New Harbinger Publications, 1992.

6 Stanford LS, Donovan ME. *Women and self-esteem*. London: Penguin, 1993.

7 Rotter JB. Generalised expectancies for internal versus external locus of control of reinforcement. *Psychological Monographs* 1966;**80**:1-28.

 8 Lazarus R. *Psychological stress and the coping process*. New York: McGraw-Hill, 1966.

 9 Watkins SJ. Improving Stockport's health. The 10th, 11th and 12th Annual Public Health Reports for Stockport 1998–2000, triennial overview. Stockport: Stockport Department of Public Health, 1998–2000.

10 MacDonald G, O'Hara K. *Ten elements of mental health, its promotion and demotion: implications for practice*. Glasgow: Society of Health Education and Health Promotion Specialists, 1998.

11 Wood J, 'The writing's on the wall', *Mental Health Occupational Therapy* (the magazine of the *Association of Occupational Therapists in Mental Health)*, March 2003.

12 Clarke S. *MAPS: an evaluation*. Stockport: Stockport Centre for Health Promotion, 2003.

8

Mainlining with *Trainspotting*: using literature to enter other worlds

CLAIRE ELLIOTT

Dr Claire Elliott, a general practitioner and tutor in medical humanities, describes the value of a contemporary novel, *Trainspotting*, in helping students and health care practitioners to make sense of a world view very different from their own. She explains how imaginative literature can help health professionals to understand patient behaviours that might initially appear senseless.

Introduction

In medical school students learn about drugs of addiction. They learn about them in pharmacology lectures between drugs for high blood pressure and drugs for asthma. They are given long lists of the pharmacological effects of drugs, both the desired effects and the side effects. In the cold light of the lecture theatre, drug-taking seems very unappealing. It is a different language from the excited one used by friends who have experimented with drugs, and some students are led to experiment themselves. Later, as doctors, it is often difficult to understand why people take drugs. Doctors have job security, affluence, and a future to think about; the attraction is a mystery. How can the excitement and the highs be worth the downsides – the urgent need for the next supply, the criminalisation, the risks of death and disease?

This chapter describes how the use of a piece of popular contemporary fiction, Irvine Welsh's *Trainspotting*,[1] can help doctors and other health care professionals to enter the world of drug addicts, and to use this alternative perspective to explore some of the vital issues. The teaching described has been used with doctors, nurses, medical students and other health professionals.

Literature and medicine: helping professionals understand their patients' worlds

Patient narratives are now recognised as a rich and important source of data in medical practice and research.[2] Nevertheless, communication between doctor and patient can be problematic. The patient tries to tell their story of illness, and the doctor then retells, and reinterprets, what s/he hears using medical language. The result is two, often conflicting, accounts of the patient's experience.[3] Health professionals are to some extent familiar with both languages but to each other usually present cases using medical constructs of illness. Moreover their familiarity with this medical construct of illness can mean that they sometimes falsely assume that the story they retell is the same as the one they have been told. The use of literature in medical education can serve two purposes here. First, it can provide a timely reminder of the differences and

'Swingeing London III' by Richard Hamilton (Screen print on paper, 1972) Images of the allure and dangers of drug taking are not new. This picture of the rock star Mick Jagger and Robert Fraser (Hamilton's gallerist at the time) is based on a press photograph from 1967 and shows the two of them handcuffed together in a police van. It exemplifies some of the glamorous and the dangerous aspects that can be associated with drug taking.

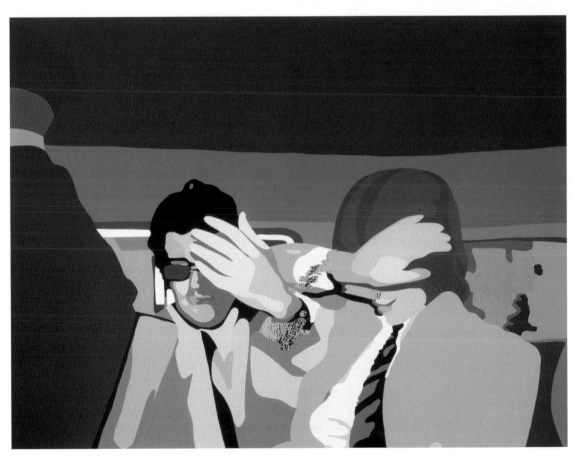

the similarities between the worlds patients and health care professionals inhabit, and second, it can facilitate understanding of the different world views these entail.

The use of literature within medicine is, of course, well established. The benefits of studying literature within medical education have a firm foundation.[4–8] Downie has identified a number of ways in which literature can be helpful to the practice of medicine, two of which are relevant to the learning objectives discussed in this chapter.[9]

Firstly, Downie feels that the treatment of the medical profession by non-medical writers is useful. Doctors have maintained their prominent position in the hierarchy of trust despite a general trend towards iconoclasm. It is easy for doctors to take their status for granted and rarely have their views and opinions challenged. Yet in the extract from *Trainspotting* discussed here, doctors – with their training and values embedded in more mainstream society – can find the values held by those they seek to help, those addicted to drugs, alien. The doctor's agenda makes no sense in the addict's world; the doctor is therefore neither trusted nor respected. The reality of daily practice supports this analysis. Doctors report that they sometimes find caring for addicts problematic, and addicts are characterised as demanding, unreliable at making and keeping appointments, and liable to make frequent requests for prescription drugs with spurious explanations of need.[10]

Secondly, Downie believes that literature can contribute to 'whole person medicine' and describes how literature can help develop an ability to perceive genuine need, the emotions and conflicts that emerge in dealing with real life, and encourage readers to more closely examine questions of morality.[9] *Trainspotting* brings out all these issues. The reader begins to feel sorry for the drug-abusing anti-hero Renton, to understand his world and to realise the problems he has had in living with his handicapped brother, his self-criticism and his alienation from society. Crucially, the reader is encouraged, through engagement with the text, to think about the values that he or she holds.

Within the realms of great Western literature, there are major works with specific relevance for the medical profession – these include *Middlemarch* by George Eliot, *The Magic Mountain* by Thomas Mann and *The Plague* by Albert Camus. There are also physician writers such as Anton Checkov, Tobias Smollett and

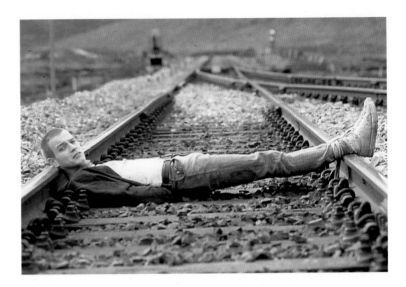

Ewan McGregor as Mark Renton on the rails in the film version of *Trainspotting*.

William Carlos Williams.[11,12] Undoubtedly, these texts are of great value to medical humanities educators but might also be daunting for the less confident reader who has little familiarity with the study of literature. Contemporary texts may help engage health care professionals who might otherwise feel inhibited by a sense that their literary insight is inadequate. Furthermore, these texts are more immediately valid when the stated objective is to provide insights into a world inhabited by their patients but nevertheless unfamiliar to many professionals.

Trainspotting: contemporary, topical and controversial

Trainspotting tells its story through the lives of four junkies, who live in Leith, near Edinburgh. The book continues to be a commercial as well as critical success, popular with many readers who do not normally buy books. It is also the most shoplifted book in Britain, and is circulated in prisons.[13] The film of the book attracted large audiences. *Trainspotting* neither glorifies nor vilifies drugs, and while it is certainly not an attempt to advocate the thrills of drug-taking, it is frank about the reasons why people do abuse drugs. As one character explains,

> Take yir best orgasm, multiply the feeling by twenty, and you're still fuckin miles off the pace. Ma dry, cracking bones are soothed and liquefied by ma heroine's tender caresses. The earth moved and it's still moving.

Yet his friends contract HIV and he nearly dies from an overdose. For Welsh, the book is about more than drug-taking *per se*:

> It's like drugs have become a whole metaphor now for consumer capitalism, the idea of chasing the high. And instant gratification, it's so much at the root of our society. It's impossible to imagine living without that.[13]

In search of a shared understanding

Trainspotting is written in a rich vernacular with phonetic spelling. This colloquial speech, which is hard for non-locals to understand, was used in the film (subtitles were added to the US version). At first, the strange and unfamiliar dialect makes *Trainspotting* hard work to read but eventually, as the reader is drawn into the dialogue, he or she begins to see the story through the eyes of the four protagonists, Renton, Begbie, Sick Boy and Spud; protagonists who feel as alienated from standard, formal English as they do from traditional life. The passage discussed in this chapter fulfils the criteria of a narrative described by Greenhalgh and Hurwitz.[14] First, it has a finite and longitudinal time sequence; a beginning, a middle and an end. Second, it assumes a story-teller and a listener whose perspectives may differ. Third, the passage deals with individuals and how they feel and think, rather than just what is done to them. Fourth, the narrative provides items of information that are not necessarily immediately relevant to the story. It offers a stark contrast to the pared-down information concerning addiction usually found in medical books. In this narrative it is the protagonist who sets the provocative agenda and not the doctor.

Parallel worlds

Trainspotting is written in disjointed and chaotic short sections, reflecting the character of an addict's life. The passage* is short enough to be read in ten minutes and can stand alone, without requiring familiarity with the entire text. One of the protagonists, Renton, reluctantly enrols on a drug rehabilitation programme, an

---

*Called 'Searching for the inner man', it is short enough to be read in ten minutes and can stand alone.

alternative to a prison sentence offered at the time of sentencing for an earlier crime. The extract involves consultations with a psychiatrist, a psychologist and a counsellor from the drug agency. The psychiatrist is probing to try to find an explanation for Renton's drug addiction within a Freudian psychoanalytic framework, whereas Renton is there only because it is obligatory. Each has their own, distinct agenda, each consistent with their own, very different, world view. Since Renton does not want to leave his drug world the exercise, drug rehabilitation, is doomed to failure.

> DR FORBES: You mention your brother, the one with the, eh, disability. The one that died. Can we talk about him? (pause)
>
> ME: Why? (pause)
>
> DR FORBES: You're reluctant to talk about your brother?
>
> ME: Naw. It's just that ah dinnae see the relevance ay that tae me being oan smack.
>
> DR FORBES: It seems that you started using heavily around the time of your brother's death.
>
> ME: A loat happened around that time. Ah'm no really sure how relevant it is tae islate ma brar's death. Ah went up tae Aberdeen at the time; the uni. Ah hated it. Then ag started oan the cross-channel ferries. Tae Holland. Access tae aw the collies ye could hope fir. (pause)
>
> DR FORBES: I'd like to go back to Aberdeen. You say you hated Aberdeen?
>
> ME: Aye.
>
> DR FORBES: What was it about Aberdeen you hated?
>
> ME: The University. The staff. The students and aw that. Ah thought they were aw boring middle-class cunts.
>
> DR FORBES: I see. You were unable to form relationships with people there.
>
> ME: No sae much unable, as unwilling, although ah suppose it means the same, for your purposes (non-committal shrug fai Dr Forbes)... ah hudnae interest in any fucker thair.*

---

*When I give the participants this extract of the book, I describe the difficulties in reading and understanding the dialect. I encourage them to read aloud in their minds which helps them to hear the language and focus on the reading. If they are stuck on any particular word, I ask them to mention this and usually someone else in the group will be able to interpret it.

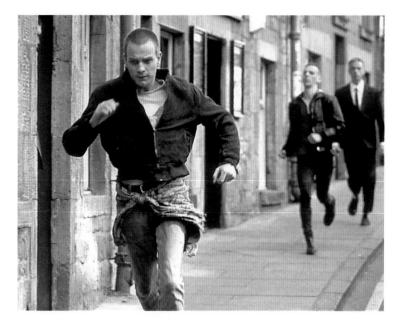

Another image from the film of *Transpotting:* here Ewan McGregor as Mark Renton and Ewen Bremner as Spud are being chased along an Edinburgh street by store detectives.

Renton's commentary on Dr Forbes makes you aware that he is only there because it is compulsory, he does not engage with him seriously ('fucked if ah could see the connection between any ay that and me takin smack').

Sometimes Renton lies, sometimes he tells the doctor only what he wants him to hear. However, Renton is inspired enough to do his own research into psychoanalysis, to interpret his own behaviour. Renton's commentary clearly indicates that he is in control, and not fitting into the stereotyped view of a drug addict. Later, he dismisses the practical behavioural approach of the clinical psychologist. Next, he meets the drug counsellor and notes that he is from a social work rather that a medical background. Renton confesses that the counsellor gets closer to understanding why he is using drugs – his failure to live up to his own and life's limitations and his subsequent alienation from society. He discusses his view of why he takes hard drugs, and whether the therapists and other professionals have the right to dissect and analyse him: 'Once ye accept that they huv that right, ye'll join them in the search fir this holy grail, this thing that makes ye tick...the dependency shifts from the drug to them'.

He has chosen to reject what they have to offer, forget the consumerism that they have opted for and, instead, choose drugs. Why, he asks, does society have to impose its values on him?

Illuminating this other world

Joanne Trautman has said that literary works can do more than simply illustrate medical subjects; they can illuminate those subjects too.[15] Before this can occur, a number of barriers to using this text must be addressed. Firstly, the colloquial language is challenging and some readers feel very alienated from it and from the characters, people they do not normally encounter and do not want to know. For others the abusive language is distasteful, and for some the difference between practising in the country and affluent areas, and practising in run-down estates of Edinburgh, adds to the sense of unfamiliarity. When these difficulties are identified and acknowledged within the larger group, it is striking how enthusiastic the readers become as they begin to discuss the extract within smaller groups. They are often keen to volunteer extracts from the text to illustrate their views, with the popular nature of the book appearing to encourage active contributions by everyone. The rich and provocative language serves to encourage a lively discussion, and a number of themes emerge as central to what *Trainspotting* seems to communicate to these readers. The themes that are expressed by readers during this teaching, and their thoughts about them, are outlined below.

A drug user's world

The addict's level of understanding and control of the situation surprise readers. Renton appears to have good insight into how the different therapists are trying to help him and the underlying theory behind their methods. Readers have commented on how Renton seems to be in charge, note that he is only attending the therapy as an alternative to prison and that he chooses, successfully, not to engage, but to dismiss the help on offer. They are impressed by Renton's analysis of the situation as he wonders whether prison might, after all, have been easier than therapy. Having researched the theories behind the therapy he is offered, Renton dismisses the psychiatrist's view that his addiction is due to an unresolved conflict with his dead handicapped brother. Interestingly, some readers felt persuaded by Renton's arguments on the futility of forcing individuals into unwanted therapy, finding themselves more sympathetic to his perspective than that of the therapists. Many, not expecting to identify with an addict, have been surprised to find they agree with Renton on a number of issues. Renton has chosen addiction over other kinds of life, in particular the one dominated by the financial rewards of work and the exhaustion that follows a busy day that many of his friends in regular employment will have. Renton dismisses the 'mortgage payments …washing machines …cars …sitting on a couch watching mind-numbing and spirit-crushing game shows, stuffing fuckin junk food intae yir mooth'. He also explains how 'junk fills the void'* which has resulted from his depression and which he feels is due to his lack of ability to change the way the world is. Some readers clearly understand his choice: at some level, their world views coincide.

The contrasting approaches used in *Trainspotting* by the psychiatrist, psychologist and drug counsellor are often raised for discussion. The psychiatrist uses a psychoanalytic method based on the medical model of addiction, the psychologist a behaviour modifying approach, and the social worker/counsellor a client-centred approach. Renton, it seems, is well aware of the differences, good and bad.

The fictional consultation

Within general practice training the consultation is the focus of much of the work.[16] Doctors are videotaped for educational and examination purposes. Emphasis is placed on language, its content and form, silences and picking up the cues from patients.[17] Looking at consultation skills is therefore a familiar technique for general practitioners, and increasingly for other practitioners.[18] In this fictional consultation, we hear the psychiatrist and Renton pass each other on different tracks. The psychiatrist persists with his own agenda and Renton (implying that the psychiatrist makes it up as he goes along), wilfully disregards any help. While some participants in seminars sympathise with the psychiatrist and feel that he is trying to make sense of Renton's life and drug habit, others feel that he is arrogant, patronising and unable to adapt his style and approach. The professional challenges raised by the fictional consultation are clear to these readers and provoke much

---

* 'Junk' is a colloquial term for heroin.

thoughtful discussion. While the intention of the workshop is not to provide answers about how to overcome problems inherent in a situation like this, it does bring the issues involved into sharp focus. The overwhelming feedback from learners concerns how much they have enjoyed and were stimulated by the seminar. They had not considered looking at fiction as a resource for learning about other worlds or seeing how others see them. Written feedback included comments such as 'It demonstrated well the insights that we can gain about people's lives' and 'It is amazing how often books can help one understand better'.

Society's perspective on drug users and their values

In *Trainspotting*, readers are presented with a powerful indictment of the prevailing values in society, values that Renton feels the rest of society is imposing on him:

> Society invents a spurious convoluted logic tae absorb and change people whae's behaviour is outside its mainstream. Suppose that ah ken aw the pros and cons, know that ah'm gaunnae huv a short life, am ay sound mind etcetera, etcetera, but still want tae use smack? They won't let you do it.

He feels the medical profession only want him to have treatment for his 'drug problem' so he will shift his dependency from drugs onto them. It is society that determines what is success or failure; he does not share their values and wonders why he should care. He asks why he is forced into rehabilitation when he wants to continue using drugs.

The ethical and legal dilemma about the legalisation of drugs is one of daily significance for many health care professionals and this extract creates a space for frank and open discussion of relevant concerns. Readers discuss the risks of using soft drugs, whether the use of hard drugs necessarily follows that of soft drugs, and whether the risks of hard drug habits are caused by the drug itself, or by its illegal status and the associated risks.

Conclusion

Stories such as that under consideration here can help health care professionals to take a tentative step into worlds which medical and pharmacological textbooks rarely evoke. By telling a story in a way that encourages the reader to engage with and think about the choices the characters make within the world in which they live, literature can provide a powerful contribution to medical education.[14] Moreover, the process of actively reading a piece of literature has many parallels to the active listening that is an essential component of a successful consultation.[19] The person's story must be heard if the communication is to be meaningful. Ann Jay, echoing the work of Robert Coles,[20] feels that as doctors we can feed our imaginations by reading fiction and engage with characters in a different way, no longer straight-jacketed by time- limited consultations, and other role-related tasks.[21] Reading and discussing this extract from *Trainspotting* provided readers with protected time to explore a view of the drug addict's world no longer centred on the medical model, but gained through stepping into a world centred on the patient.

Acknowledgement

My thanks to David Misselbrook with whom I originally planned a seminar using *Trainspotting*.[22]

References

1 Welsh I. *Trainspotting*. London: Vintage, 1999.

2 Greenhalgh T. Narrative based medicine in an evidence based world. In: Greenhalgh T, Hurwitz B (eds). *Narrative based medicine*. London: BMJ Books, 1998.

3 Hunter KM. *The doctors' stories*. Princeton, New Jersey: Princeton University Press, 1991.

4 Hunter KM, Charon R, Coulehan JL. The study of literature in medical education. *Acad Med* 1995:**70**;787–94.

5 Jones AH. Literature and medicine: an evolving canon. *Lancet* 1996; **348**:1360–62.

6 McLellan MF, Jones AH. Why literature and medicine? *Lancet* 1996; **348**:109–11.

7 Charon R, Trautmann Banks J, Connelly JE, Hawkins AH *et al.* Literature and medicine: contributions to clinical practice. *An Int Med* 1995;**122**: 599–606.

8   Kirklin D, Meakin R, Singh S *et al*. Living with and dying from cancer: a humanities special study module. *J Med Ethics: Medical Humanities* 2000;**26**:51–4.

9   Downie RS. Literature and medicine. *J Med Ethics* 1991; **17**:93–96, 98.

10 Davies A, Huxley P. Survey of general practitioners' opinions on treatment of opiate user. *BMJ* 1997;**314**:1173.

11 McLellan MF. Literature and medicine: some major works. *Lancet* 1996;**349**:1014–16.

12 McLellan MF. Literature and medicine: physician-writers. *Lancet* 1997 **349**:564–671.

13 O'Shea W, Shapiro D. Interview with Irvine Welsh, *Feed*, 9 March 1999.

14 Greenhalgh T, Hurwitz B, 'Why study narrative?' In: Greenhalgh T, Hurwitz B (eds). *Narrative based medicine*. London: BMJ Books, 1998.

15 Trautmann J. The wonders of literature and medicine. In: Self D (ed). *The role of the humanities in medical education*. Norfolk, VA: Teagle and Little, 1978.

16 Pendleton D, Schofield T, Tate P, Havelock P. *The consultation: an approach to learning and teaching*. Oxford: OUP, 1984.

17 Neighbour R. *The inner consultation: how to develop an effective and intuitive consulting style*. Newbury: Petroc Press, 1999.

18 Kurtz S, Silverman J. The Calgary-Cambridge Observation Guides: an aid to defining the curriculum and organising the teaching in communication training programmes. *Med Educ* 1996;**30**:83–9.

19 Tate P. *The doctor's communication handbook*. Abingdon: Radcliffe Medical Press, 1994.

20 Cole R. *The call of stories: teaching and the moral imagination*. Boston: Houghton Mifflin, 1989.

21 Jay A. A personal response to: *The woman who walked into doors* by Roddy Doyle. *J Med Ethics: Medical Humanities* 2000;**26**:58–9.

22 Elliott C, Misselbrook D. Escape or instruction? A description of a seminar for general practitioners on medicine and literature. *J Med Ethics: Medical Humanities* 2002;**28**:53–4.

9

The tattooed intruder: in search of a healing environment

MICHELE PETRONE

Artist Michele Petrone relates a dream in which he confronted not only his cancer, but also the alienation and powerlessness he experienced as a hospital patient. His commentary describes what he learned from writing about this dream, from sharing it with others, and suggests its potential value to those working in health care settings.

The tattooed intruder tells the story of a nightmare I had whilst in hospital receiving treatment for Hodgkin's disease. It is reproduced here in full and followed by a commentary in which I explain what I learnt from writing this piece, and what I believe health care practitioners and health service providers have to learn from my experience. Although the story told is mine, the experiences recounted will, I suspect, be familiar to many patients and families.

The tattooed intruder

'Shit!' Startled in my sleep. Towering above me, beside my bed, was this tattooed stranger. Menacing crude indigo tattoos on his scrawny-yellowed skin. Not pictorial, but almost as if self-inflicted, drunken inked scratchings, piercings, mainly on his neck. I remembered particularly this large square, amongst others, over his Adam's apple, his voice box. Who was he? What was he doing standing over me? I don't know him. He scares me.

I awake. It's the middle of the night. It's 4am. I call for a urine bottle. I'm on a fluid chart so all my pee has to be measured and my last one is full. It gives me a chance to wake fully, pull out my notebook to not forget this nightmare and write it down. How could I forget it? But like a dream startled in the night, this was the one I wanted to have forgotten about in the morning.

I know who he is. He is my cancer. The tattooed intruder. He has no name. Only a description. Yet he is a part of me that I don't recognise. That is what brings tears to my eyes. In the calm darkness. In the stillness of the night emerges death. I want to think it is only a shadow, a sign, a symbol, a possibility. Not a fact this time. But it is a possibility I am aware of. A possibility I want to deny. Another throat-cracked, teeth-clenched, sick stomach, body-shuddering tear swells in my eyes. Blurring my vision.

I continue to write in this emotional haze, through this painful sea, that threatens to drown me. Yet I have this sleep-walking drive to ink the tattoo here on this paper. Unthought, uncorrected, just scrawled as it is, gripped in my tracks. Word for word, moment for moment, tear beat, heart shudder. This is no premonition. No dream to be forgotten in the morning. This is what is happening.

As my senses are fully taking in, I'm in the dimly lit corner of a four-bedded ward. The sound of the twenty-four hour constant fungal extractor is the measure of my silence. I remember I am tethered, to a LCD-flashing chemo pump beside my bed, by the triple alumen Hickman line that protrudes out from a gash in my chest, still only two days sore and the black dissolving stitches still visible. The red electronic display flashing in three descending lines, like those of a mobile phone on charge. Only it is a sign of me being charged day and night by the cisplatin chemotherapy drug and accompanying saline solution. Charging through my body. 0.50 mls per hour and 0.48 mls per hour respectively. What is that 0.02 mls difference, flush? Who knows. 0.02 mls dash of healing.

I have nausea on the tip of my throat, standing at the entrance of my gut. And a constant ache round my temples. It is not as bad as times before. But it is a sickness I did not feel three days ago, before my treatment started. This is not my bedroom of three days ago either. I know it is now my home. Three different, institution-patterned curtains

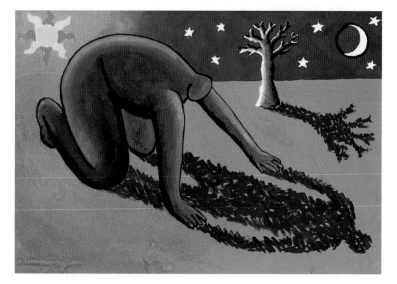

'Shadow' by Michele Angelo Petrone
As in the dream, my cancer forced me to face my shadow, the darker side to life, death, my fear that I may die from the cancer. Actually I now realise that we all die eventually, and that death is not a failure but a part of life. It is still frightening. It is our mortality which underlies the diagnosis of any life-threatening disease.

partition me from three other beds, and from the outside ward. Behind me on my left, someone else is also awake. He frightens me also. I know his name. But we haven't spoken. His white patchy skin, scrawny skeleton, cowered bent-forth stance from which hang his pyjamas stalk me. Tell-tale signs of future possible side effect of my impending transplant. Graft versus host disease. Common enough here as people talk about it in the corridors, by the nurses in its abbreviated terms GVHD. One of the many acronyms... HGL (Hodgkin's lymphoma – my disease), NHGL (non-Hodgkin's), AML (acute myeloid leukaemia).

GVHD. That haunts me. Because that is not real for me yet, and may not be. But it haunts me because of its possibility, because of my decision. Because of a frightening possible side effect of my decision. A decision to go ahead with this bone marrow transplant from my Italian cousin. She is a perfect match. But she is not my bone marrow. And so there is a chance that her bone marrow, once transplanted into my body, through what is now a relatively simple procedure – a blood transfusion after enforced growth of her stem cells through injections, and harvesting through transfusion – may reject my body. They say it can be chemically, medically controlled. But I can see his skin has been rejected. He looks half ghost, the patches of pigment less, bloodless, lifeless, what do I call it, engulfing his body.

I didn't realise until yesterday morning that the boy in the other window is also suffering from this. Latex gloves cover his raw skinless hands. His girlfriend explained that he now has GVHD in his liver and is in day care receiving the drug to combat this. And he is still smiling. No let up since 1998 for him, except for one holiday, a cruise, to find out after this that he had relapsed again with non-Hodgkin's lymphoma. His bed is empty but is always here for him. His bag keeps watch beside it, a constant reminder, that a bed awaits for when he is more ill. Everyday he returns for five minutes, ten minutes, half an hour. A quick hello. 'I'm going home,' he says cheerfully. 'Just waiting for my blood test.' And off he goes with his girlfriend, who bears a T-shirt with 'Treat me like a princess' on it. She smiles too, disbelieving of his constant outward cheerful demeanour that hides a myriad of constant disappointments and hardships.

Here you can't but be confronted by future side effects, sickness, decisions, enforced, unknown, unwanted, even agreed to. I'm still one of the well ones. I still have my hair, my short goatee stubble, my slight tan from my recent Italian holiday. I pass open doors with people, bald, ashen, gaunt, slumped in chairs, silent, alone, waiting for it all to be over. Room after room. Surrounded not by personally picked paraphernalia of homely delights. No individual swathes of taste, neither Habitat nor Ikea, neither Harrods nor World of Leather. But hospital property, polystyrene ceiling tiles, miles of tasteless curtain track, the obligatory visitor's chair by every metal institutional bed. The fan, the blood pressure pump stand. The oxygen mask and the green tubes. The angle-poise lamp. The bed number, the room number, the ward number, the floor number. The alarm switches, the fluorescent light switches. The sickness bowls. The definitely not bedroom-carpeted lino floors. The alcohol wipes. The functional sinks. The weighing scales and the sharps-only bins. The communal telly, the hospital clock. The smoke alarm and tell-tale security, safety indicators. Left, right, up, down and all around. And yet it feels safe.

I want to go to sleep now. I want to go to the loo but I remember that my loo is the plastic bottle with its 'ml' counters up its side. A fan swathes some coolish air on my face, a somewhat short relief from the constant fresh less-heated environment. I may need a cool drink too. It's a hassle. My tethered lead doesn't allow my free movement. A metre or two to the left or right of the bed. I could unplug for a moment or two, wheel my five unoiled screeching castors around to waken my other room companion. The only one asleep, too sick to be awake. I'm reminded of an Antoine de Saint-Exupéry quote that the beauty of the desert is that it conceals a well. Oh where is that fucking well?

Author's commentary

It was cathartic to write this down… I was literally recalling a dream, a nightmare on the ward at 4am. Written just after waking, the writing helped me to gather my feelings and emotions, to identify my fears and my concerns, to recognise where I was and how I was. It is really hard to be able to express your feelings in the hospital environment and even though the dream was startling, frightening, it helped me place myself, express myself to myself, and that was such a release.

Let me explain what it was like, what it must be like for so many others.

I am in a shared ward, with people I have never met before. No one introduces us; you introduce yourselves, if you have the strength. A sudden intimacy, with a room full of strangers. All of them not well, some dying. Can you imagine that, dying in a room with people you have never met before?

The struggle to get well, to live, is impacted by ridiculous things, such as a communal television. I want it turned off, I want silence, but another person wants to drown the ticking of time, with its loud monotony. We all have our different ways, and now we have to struggle between us.

Funny also how in hospital the people who are ill are not trusted. Firstly with our medication – at home it is OK, here not. And then if I have to take *my* hospital notes with me, they are sealed in a big brown envelope. Why am I, why are we, not trusted?

Everything is decided for us, when we are woken, when the light goes out, when we eat, and what we are offered to eat; everything.

The hospital environment is not homely, and not intended to be homely methinks, how could it be? Can a hospital environment be a healing environment? I think this possibility is something that is hugely overlooked. I am not talking hygiene and cleanliness. I am talking beauty and peace, about how soothing looking out onto a garden with trickling water can be.

But the worst thing for me is privacy. Not being able to have intimate moments with my partner, private conversations with my friends. Having my own room made such a difference. Can you imagine trying to talk to the doctors and nurses on the ward round about the serious side effects of the transplant, with only a flimsy curtain between that conversation and those same side effects being so graphically, so physically, expressed by my co-ward patients? I wasn't able to have that conversation in this environment and so days passed, with all of these unanswered questions and unexpressed fears and frustrations bottled inside, before a nurse told me I could request a consultation in a private room, away from the open ward.

The truth is – BEING IN A HOSPITAL IS FRIGHTENING. The impact of being in an institutionalised environment, away from home, with no privacy, power or control, is immense. For me, although it was hard to write the nightmare up, it was the eye of the storm. The writing enabled me to talk through those issues, particularly the impact on me of living so closely with other patients suffering serious side effects of the transplant that was proposed for me. And then *The tattooed intruder* became the basis of my questions to my consultant. I probably wouldn't have asked my consultant about all of the issues I did if it wasn't for my dream. A dream born of the less than perfect environment I had found myself in. In turn, the answers I received gave me more confidence about the treatment I was to receive. Funny how these things work.

Acknowledgement

Some material in this chapter first appeared in Petrone M. The tattooed intruder. *J Med Ethics: Medical Humanities* 2002;**28**:29. It is reproduced here by kind permission of the BMJ Publishing Group.

10

Instinct and effort: caring for an ill child

MICHAEL ROWE

Dr Michael Rowe examines the impact his son Jesse's fatal illness had
on Jesse himself, on his family, and on Michael as both parent and health
care professional. Writing has enabled him better to understand the
experience, and to articulate what he has learnt as a practitioner
concerning the human needs of patients and families in such a
predicament.

My son Jesse died in 1995, at age nineteen, after a three-month
hospitalisation that started with a liver transplant. Since his death
I have talked with many parents and others about my experiences
with Jesse, and in doing so I have detected what I think are two
related beliefs about parenting. The first is that good parents
possess a bottomless well of love for their children. The second is
that the efforts they make on their children's behalf flow from that
well. While parents often commiserate with each other around
their troublesome, unruly children and the never-ending work of
caring for them, there is a tongue-in-cheek quality to such
complaints, a subtext that says, 'None of this effort amounts to
much for parents who love their children'. Parents and those who
observe them never hold these two beliefs more strongly than
when children fall seriously ill.

Two problems may follow from allegiance to these beliefs. The
first is the guilt that parents feel when exhaustion sets in, that is,
when effort really is effort. The second is that some doctors view
parents – by virtue of their parental roles – as essentially irrational.
The belief of doctors and others in a bottomless well of parental
love, which might be called parental instinct, leads them to

discount or ignore the 'effort' side of caregiving, since effort, by its nature, has its peaks and its valleys, its beginnings and its ends. Thus the triumph of parents who care for an ill child in a tangle of their love, instinct, and effort, and continue to find a way to fight and witness for their child, goes unacknowledged and is banished from thought. This lack of recognition and acknowledgment denies parents the small comfort it might have offered when, sadly, all effort comes to naught.

All this is too broadly stated; a problem I hope to correct after introducing Jesse and telling three brief stories about my relationship with him. In addition, my theme does not address the fact that some parents think doctors and other health professionals treat them as caretakers rather than caregivers. These parents feel that doctors view them as mere dispensers, on command, of facts and symptoms that the doctor can, in turn, translate into clinical information. Nor does my theme address the involvement of children in decision making about their own care. My theme is intentionally narrower. I wish to examine the tension that exists between parental instinct, which I define roughly as natural and unquestioned reactions and responses to a threat to the child's health or safety, and which I equate roughly with parental love, and effort, which I define roughly as intentional acts, with intended ends, for the child's sake.

Jesse

Jesse Harlan-Rowe was born in 1975 in New Haven, Connecticut. Between the ages of three and seventeen months he had three operations for hydrocephalus, a condition in which the ventricles – spaces in the brain that produce and house cerebrospinal fluid which cushions the brain – are unable to drain their excess fluid into the blood. The ventricles grow, squeezing the brain and causing lethargy and projectile vomiting. Without medical intervention the child may die at an early age. Surgery for hydrocephalus involves inserting a metal shunt through the back of the skull, connecting a thin plastic tube to the shunt, and threading the tube under the skin and down to the abdominal cavity where it drains off the excess fluid. After the third operation, Jesse was in remission for the rest of his life, though he went through reams of paper drawing caricatures of big-headed males.

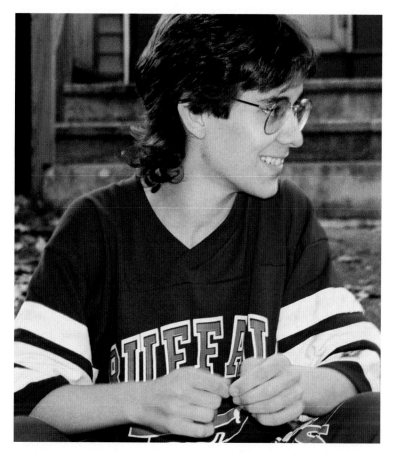

Jesse Harlan-Rowe, just before his nineteenth birthday, in the fall of 1994 on the front steps of our house. My sister took this photo. I used to hate the ritual of end-of-visit photo taking, but now I submit happily. This is my favourite photo of Jesse.

Jesse's medical problems resurfaced in adolescence. In 1991, at age fifteen, he was diagnosed with ulcerative colitis, a serious intestinal disease. In 1992 he was diagnosed with a mild case of sclerosing cholangitis, a scarring and narrowing of the bile ducts going into the liver. In 1993 he had surgery for colitis. An arteriogram performed shortly before that operation, however, revealed early-stage cirrhosis of the liver. In 1994, Jesse was wait-listed for a liver transplant at a hospital in New York City. In early May 1995 he received a liver transplant. All seemed well at first, but four days after transplant he was taken back into surgery with a rising fever and severe stomach pain. His surgeons found they had inadvertently perforated his intestine while cutting through scar tissue that had built up after his colitis surgery in 1993. They sewed up the perforation, but peritonitis had already set in and was followed swiftly by sepsis and multi-organ failure. Against all expectations, Jesse rallied and received a second liver transplant in early June.

Two weeks later another perforation, this time a result of his weak-ened condition, was found during another surgery, and another bout of sepsis followed. Again he rallied, but a final downturn and another bout of sepsis occurred. He died in early August 1995 after a total of thirteen operations, including two liver transplants and a splenectomy.

Jesse was a talented artist. He was quiet and withdrawn but had a fine wit when he did talk. He was fiercely loyal to a few close friends, to athletes whose bodies did not betray them, to his favorite comic book artists, and to superheroes of myth and popular culture. There was a vulnerability about him that many seemed to respond to with a quiet protectiveness, a 'looking out for'. He rarely talked about himself or his fears about his medical problems, though we never stopped trying to get him to do that. And he was strong in a quiet way that fooled me for a long time, so quiet, so little disposed to asserting himself or his needs, that you might think he couldn't fight for himself. Not true. I think, now, that he saw himself as one of the superheroes or ancient warriors he admired, and his struggle with illness as one element in the quest saga of his life.

Three stories

My first story concerns an incident from the fall of 1978, around the time of Jesse's third birthday. His mother, Rachel,* and I were in the midst of early-separation chaos, with first I, then she, then I, moving out of our apartment in New Haven, Connecticut. Jesse stayed in the apartment, at the centre of our chaos but at least not having to move with it. At the time of this story, Jesse would go with Rachel in the morning to the preschool where she taught, and I would pick him up after work or she would bring him back to the apartment after I got home. One evening I was standing by the doorway separating the kitchen and dining room when Jesse came running from the kitchen and tripped and fell at the point where the linoleum floor of the kitchen met the dining-room carpet. I turned, grabbed, picked him up, and asked him if he was all right before I knew what I was doing.

---

*This, like the names of all characters other than Jesse in this chapter, is a pseudonym.

'Aha!' I thought. 'So it's not maternal instinct, after all. It's parental instinct!'

It's not that I had been what I would call a neglectful father. Rachel and I had been strong together for Jesse, exciting the admiration of his doctors and nurses, during the first year and a half of his life and three operations for hydrocephalus. After that crisis passed, though, I became absorbed in my work while Rachel stayed home and was the main nurturing presence in Jesse's life. Thus the Eureka! effect for me, a first-time father, of my 'instinctive' response to his fall on the dining room carpet that day.

The second story concerns an incident in May 1993. I had remarried and Jesse now had a younger brother and sister. Two years earlier he had been diagnosed with ulcerative colitis. Steroids and other drugs failed to bring it under control. It was May 1993, two months away from colitis surgery and, though we didn't know it at the time, from diagnosis of early-stage cirrhosis of the liver. Jesse was seeing Dr Oran, a haematologist, for a bone-marrow biopsy, one of a number of tests aimed at determining the cause of his enlarged spleen. Dr Oran was kind and thorough in explaining the procedure. He made only one mistake, but it was a big one. He told Jesse the procedure wouldn't hurt.

Jesse took off his pants, placed a paper apron over his legs, and sat at the edge of the examining table, as instructed. Dr Oran came back in and had him lie on his left side with his legs curled up. Dr Oran then took a long thick needle and slowly pushed it through the skin to a vertebra in his lower back, through the vertebra and into the marrow, where he extracted a tiny sample of that life-giving substance. Jesse winced hard and let out a small groan. After it was over he got dressed, slowly.

'It hurt. A lot.'

Outside, we sat in the car in the parking lot behind the medical building. I looked at the white aluminum-sided three-storey houses in front of us beyond the parking lot fence.

'Dr Oran was wrong to tell you it wouldn't hurt.' And, I felt, I was wrong not to have warned him that it would or to reprove Dr Oran for his remark.

Shrug, a mournful nod.

'Tell you what, we'll stop and get something to eat on the way back home. Whatever you want.'

Little smile.

'Where would you like to go?'

'I don't know. Anywhere is fine.'

But he had a bad 'accident' of diarrhoea on the way to the restaurant. I reassured him that it didn't bother me, that it wasn't his fault, all the flapdoodle one has to say and all of which is true, but none of which can cover the other's shame for having lost control at the place where privacy and dignity coexist. We got home. I put my jacket around him and shooed everyone away. We went downstairs to the washing machine. I found him some clean clothes. I felt badly for him, but never felt more like a father, his protector, than I did at that moment.

Thinking of this incident later on, I asked myself why this event filled me with such sorrow, given all that Jesse went through in his life and all the times I'd been with him for other procedures and office visits and blood draws. And filled me with such sweet propinquity. It's true that the bone marrow biopsy was one of the most painful and least sedated of all procedures Jesse had outside of the hospital. Then again, it involved an invasion of his spinal column, a fearful enough procedure for any parent but one that reminded me of the unruly watery cushions over his brain – the ventricles that had failed to drain their excess cerebrospinal fluid properly. Or was it Jesse's need, and my desire to protect him, that moved me, and maybe the recognition that I had hit the right notes with him, and we had hit the right notes together?[1]

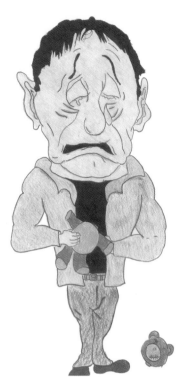

Jesse drew this (in colour in the original) when he was about 17. At a glance, it's just a simple caricature of a silly old man (or is he a boy wearing an old man's mask?) crying over a broken teddy bear. Yet ridiculous as he is, his sorrow is heartbreaking, even terrifying, too.

The third story concerns an insight I had four years after Jesse's death while working on a book about him. I wrote about going back to the hospital to call memory from its cave, reentering the admissions area from the back end and reversing the path Jesse and I had taken on 5 May 1995 when he was admitted to wait for his transplant. I wrote about turning back when I reached the waiting room, perhaps because I wasn't sure what I would say if the receptionist asked, 'Can I help you?' meaning, What was I doing there if I was not sick myself or bringing in someone who was? What would I say? That this was the place where we sat on the couches for an hour trying to be nonchalant about why we were sitting there? That just around the corner in a tiny airless room I had sat with Jesse as we signed permission for surgery that might save his life or end it? And that I just wanted to relive those

148

moments? 'And effort,' I wrote, 'stops somewhere, even with one's child.' This comment would have made more sense in connection with other efforts I made on Jesse's behalf, but regardless of its reference point, it shocked me as I set it down.

Discussion

The first of my three stories involves an initiation into a new level of parenthood, a recognition that I had the right stuff to be a parent because I had acted in a way I thought any good parent should – selflessly, focused only on Jesse's needs. The third story, ending, in effect, with the thought that instinct alone does not make a good parent, involves my acknowledgment of another initiation, into another level of parenthood, an initiation that had already taken place somewhere during the months and years of taking Jesse to hundreds of doctor's visits, blood draws, and medical procedures, strategising with his doctors, and Jesse's mother, Rachel, and my wife, Gail, making friends with the insurance coordinator at our health plan, anything that might give Jesse a toehold on a sheer cliff. The second story involves my sense of rightness in my relationship with Jesse and my care of him that day, whether that care emerged from instinct or effort.

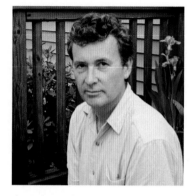

The author, spring 2002.

Most parents love their children and want good things for them, even if their own needs, failed ambitions, and other personal idiosyncrasies and upbringings may complicate their love. Parents who do much for their children during relatively untroubled times do more for them when they are seriously ill. They expect this of themselves as society expects it of them. Those who are better educated, or have done more research on their child's condition, or can converse more easily with doctors, are seen as good parents whose skills come into play secondarily. They may also be seen as meddlesome and oppositional to the doctor's authority. Parenting, then, can be described as a 'master status,' one that trumps or absorbs other statuses such as education, occupation, and other factors that shape parents' care for their children.

Because of the perceived centrality of the parenting instinct, the hard work involved in caring for an ill child receives less attention than it should. In fact, parents draw on their love and instinct, their conscious learning and effort, their intellect and strategy, even their willingness to set aside the promptings of love in order to see what they have missed, or to do what they had not considered doing before. Parents leave no stone unturned in their survey of people and resources that might point to, or make possible, the one act that can save their child's life. In addition, a focus on instinct misses the point that the labour of love is the hardest labour of all. Just ask your mother. It is the effort parents make which does not simply flow from love or instinct that merits our admiration. Parents, it seems, can never do enough, and all they do may still fall short of what is needed.

The split between our deepest feelings and conscious efforts is played out in the doctor–parent relationship. In simplified form, it goes something like this. Doctors, often parents themselves, have all the feelings of parents, but hold these feelings back in an effort to maintain their objectivity. Parents want doctors to be technically competent but compassionate as well, to have an inkling of their child's suffering and their own, but often don't sense this compassion in the doctors caring for their child. Doctors expect to see parental instinct in parents and conflate it with the efforts they see parents make. When such dynamics are at work, doctors and parents are not so much ships passing in the night as ships together in a fog that keeps them from seeing each other clearly. Parents need doctors to recognise the whole person that every parent is: a loving, sometimes panicked, sometimes fiercely calculating parent; an adult; a worker; and the person willing to bring all of himself, or herself, to bear on the one thing that now matters in the world—the health and safety of the child. Such recognition of the person behind the parent might shift the interaction between parent and doctor in a subtly different direction and might clear away some of the fog that stops parents and doctors from seeing each other clearly.

When medical and parental efforts fail to heal the child, parents, who must live with the knowledge that effort and love were not enough, might experience just a bit less guilt over the child that died if there were open acknowledgement of the important role that parental love *and* parental effort, together, play in the care of their child. This acknowledgement might also reduce parental guilt about surviving children, whom parents now understand they cannot protect from the vagaries of luck or fate. Perhaps, too, parents might be a bit less inclined to engage in the recriminations and distancings that can come between spouses

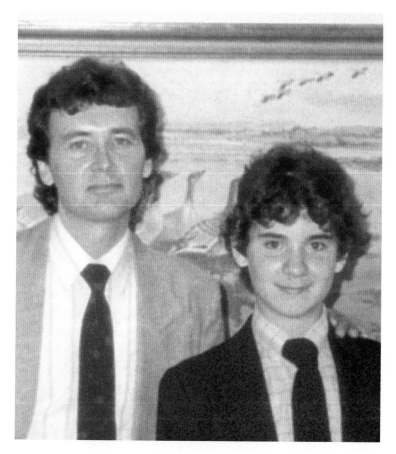

The author with Jesse, age thirteen, 1989, at a showing of the wildlife drawings of the author's father. A videotape of this event shows Jesse, animated, talking with his grandfather's friends, a surprise for the memory of those who were close to this shy (then) child.

after a child's death. And perhaps this is hoping for far too much. In the end all parents have their own ways of coping, their own honesties and evasions and ways of being in the world. As parents, we cannot always see the effects of our honesty and evasions on those around us. Yet facing the limitations of our efforts, while acknowledging the reach of them, can be a source of strength, not weakness, for others, including our children, who look to us to learn how they might be in the world.

The psychologically minded reader may have guessed by now that I protest too much. I, too, see my love for my son as a bottomless well. I, too, feel not only that effort should have felt like no effort at all, but also that one or the other or both – love or effort – should have been enough to see Jesse through. I have erred on the side of effort in order to make my point. Instinct and conscious effort do not stand at opposite poles. My love for my son, my parental instinct, my social and cultural learning about what good

151

parents do, my own sense of myself, were fuel for my efforts and reminders that I must not stray from the path of caring when effort weighed me down. My desire to be a good parent when Jesse was three years old found a way to tell me I possessed as much instinct to protect him as any mother would, and this new sense of myself helped me learn how to take care of him. Over time, giving that care, along with the knowledge that I did care deeply, allowed me to see that neither love nor instinct dictated or guaranteed this giving. If I finally had to let go of the illusion of love that brooks no resistance, I could also see that I strove to bring all of myself into the fray to be good for Jesse.

Conclusion

Caring for an ill child is one form of parenting as it is one form of human relationship, with its own characteristics and differences, especially those involving the awesome power of the caregiver. It is a form of the 'health care relationship', the one in which ill children spend more time than they do in relationships with their doctors.[2] The health care relationship of parents and children also involves their health care relationships with doctors and nurses. In these relationships parents, subject to the influences of experience and learning and inner need, draw on their minds and hearts to make decisions in the best interests of their children when those children are not of an age, or not in a condition, to make such decisions for themselves. Both doctors and parents would do well to honour those efforts made in the name of love.

References

1   I tell this story in a slightly different form in my memoir, *The book of Jesse: A story of youth, illness, and medicine.* Washington, DC: The Francis Press, 2002.
2   See Kleinman A. *The illness narratives: suffering, healing, and the human condition.* New York: Basic Books, 1988.

11

Poetry and caring: healing the within

JOHN FOX

Poetry therapist John Fox offers a compelling account of the healing power of creative expression for all those affected by illness – patients, those who love them, and the professionals who care for them.

There lives the dearest freshness deep down things

   – Gerard Manley Hopkins

I'm a spiritual person and writing poetry is increasingly important to me in my work. When you work with thousands of children with cancer over 30 odd years – more than half of whom have died – you have to confront certain issues. Poetry has helped me make sense of things.

   – John Graham-Pole, MD, Professor of Pediatrics at the
      University of Florida at Gainesville, Shands Hospital

What I want to consider in this chapter is poetry and healing. That is, the potential of our words and the words of others, *intentionally used*, to enhance a patient's experience of the *healing environment* and help both patient and hospital personnel make contact with what I am going to call 'the within'.

How could the language of poetry heal the within? What *is* the 'within?' How could our words, even when we are confronted with illness and circumstances of illness that are painful and heart-breaking, help us to speak what is true, help us to listen?

The poet Muriel Rukeyser has said that the universe is not really made up of atoms, it's made up of stories. In the course of this chapter, I will introduce the voices of physicians, nurses and patients who have been helped by poetry and creative writing. They will share their stories and address questions about how poetry heals. My own story, of how I came to be a poetry therapist, will serve as a brief introduction to the rest of the chapter.

Meeting the challenges of a difficult world

Beyond our attempts to 'cure' or 'solve' particular problems, communicating truth in the lines of a healing poem helps to foster a courageous spirit. Expression of one's creative voice can aid a person in meeting the challenge of a difficult world.

I have found, in 18 years of work as a poetry therapist and a lifetime of being a lover of words, that people, when treated with deep respect and curiosity, write poetry that can reveal a wholeness; a spirit rooted in integrity, simplicity and a sense of compassion. Integrating these basic, foundational qualities will help sustain people in the midst of incredible crises, illness, painful experiences and challenging life transitions.

We strengthen the whole healing process by remembering and communicating creatively the essential character and original nature of who we are.

I know this not only as a poetry therapist but also as a patient. I remember a poem I wrote at 18 as I was confronting the amputation of my right leg below the knee. I had for years dealt with the problem – the result of a genetic disorder – of neurofibromatosis. Poetry had become my way of not only naming what my experience was during numerous hospital visits and surgeries – but also of remembering the larger world, in which I was, in spite of my physical problem, an enthusiastic participant.

But at that time in my life, during such a crisis, poetry was also a companion in the dark. What I discovered was that my poems sometimes gave me insights; startling insights I would not have had if I hadn't bothered to write. My poems, while allowing me to state the truth of what troubled me, also insisted that I pay attention to my life.

That receptivity made a difference because it required that I consider not only what I experienced in relationship *to* my life but also what life was bringing to me. I wrote one such poem shortly after I visited my doctor.

IN THE HOSPITAL WAITING ROOM

There was a child went forth every day,
And the first object he looked upon, that object he became.
And that object became part of him for the day or a certain part
    of the day,
Or for many years or stretching cycles of years.

    – Walt Whitman

The people are seated in the chairs, lined
in the halls and waiting:
some looking at Time, most somber:
save two little girls, patient
and singing – one's embroidering,
a singing embroidery!

Waiting for nothing, skipping along
past the people, past office partitions
that are not there for these little children,
so much like garden-walkers!

Whitman, I go forth, yet, shall I become
pictures of my bones?
X-rayed through this dense sea, this film shows me
the heavy anchor that I seem to be.
This goes deepest.

Behind the picture is light!

I had seen many, many X-rays in my life, since about age five, all of
my leg with its deformities and problems. The stanza of Whitman's
poem, 'There was a child went forth', seemed so appropriate for
naming what I had had to deal with.

Yet, the tension I felt between the joyful children in the waiting
room and the sombre adults – and the tension within myself –
shook me to ask the hard question I did. What I noticed might
sound odd or simplistic but the very fact that it was *light* that
shone through that X-ray of my wounded bones, came to me, at
eighteen, as a revelation.

That insight was not the end of my struggle. There was plenty
of my journey left that included periods of near despair. But that
poem did act as a beacon during those darker times.

The history of poetry therapy

In the late eighteenth century, noted physician Benjamin Rush introduced poetry as a form of therapy at Pennsylvania Hospital in Philadelphia. We don't know what form 'poetry therapy' took at that time, and history tells us that the treatment of individuals in mental hospitals was frequently ignorant, even brutal, but the use of poetry is an indication that from a very early time more enlightened doctors like Rush recognised the power of words to heal. Rush said of poets that they 'view the human mind in all its operations, whether natural or morbid, with a microscopic eye, and hence many things arrest their attention, which escape the notice of physicians'. Over 200 years later, poetry therapy is still employed at Pennsylvania Hospital.

Walt Whitman tended wounded soldiers during the American Civil War, reading poetry to them on hospital wards and in the field. He wrote and read poems about the grief of war, courage and the human aspects of a soldier's life. The use of libraries in hospitals grew immensely during World War I, as wounded veterans sought out words for solace and healing. The poems of Wilfred Owen, Rupert Brooke, Siegfried Sassoon, ee cummings and Robert Graves all expressed war's horror and uselessness – and stood as a witness for other veterans to what they had also experienced.

In the late 1920s, a Brooklyn pharmacist named Eli Greifer offered 'poetic prescriptions' to people filling their drug prescriptions. In 1928, Greifer opened the 'Remedy Rhyme Gallery' in Greenwich Village. Greifer believed that memorisation of poems was useful for a process of healing he called 'psychosurgery'. He felt it was possible to 'psychograft' the thoughts and feelings of great people into one's own psyche. Poems by Keats, Wordsworth and Blake were used as part of his 'apothecary'.

Methodologies of poetry therapy have developed extensively since Greifer's time, and in discussing his 'psychografting' memorisation technique, he sounds more shaman than pharmacist:

> We have here no less than a psychograft by memorization in the inmost reaches of the brain, where the soul can allow the soul-stuff of stalwart poet-prophets to 'take' and to become one with the spirit of the patient. Here is insight. Here is introjection. Here is ennoblement of the spirit of man – by

blood transfusing the personality with the greatest insights of all the greatest souled poets of all ages… beautiful figures of speech, the melody of rhythm and meter and assonance… painted scenes… dramatic episodes, love's pervasiveness – all are consecrated by the master poets to gently enter and transfuse the ailing subconscious, the abraded and suffering personality.[1]

In 1958, Greifer met Dr Jack Leedy, the directing psychiatrist at Cumberland Hospital in Brooklyn. It was an auspicious meeting for the future of poetry therapy. Leedy, ignoring the disdain of many psychiatric and medical colleagues, became an ardent advocate for the use of poetry in therapy. He was, through his compassion, charm and drive, a major force in bringing the use of poetry to the attention of the mental health profession.

Many others besides Leedy and Greifer have done important pioneering work in this healing art since the mid-1950s. Sherry Reiter, an early colleague of Jack Leedy, recalls an historic milestone of the poetry therapy movement:

By 1980 poetry therapy as a healing tool was flourishing in different parts of the United States. I contacted everyone we knew interested in poetry and healing and invited them to a conference held at the New School for Social Research in New York City, the place I had earlier taught courses with Dr Leedy. We met in order to become the National Association for Poetry Therapy.

In 1981, the Association further developed professional standards for ethics, training and certification/registration. Membership is international with practitioners and interested people throughout the world including the UK, Ireland, Italy, Lithuania, Israel, Canada, Japan, Greece and Germany. It comprises a wide-range of professional disciplines, schools of therapy, educational affiliations, artistic domains, and other fields of training in both psychology and medicine.

Poetry therapy uses the intentional writing and reading of poetry by a trained biblio-, poetry or journal therapist to further therapeutic goals and enhance the well-being of individuals and groups through the integration of emotional, cognitive, spiritual and social aspects of self.

An act of human magic

The ritual chants and incantations of shamanism, the healing songs and magic of primitive people with their rich core of poetry, illustrate the vital role of art in ancient medicine. Poetry is indeed a force, an act of human magic, that alters the way we see our lives and so changes us.

– Morris R Morrison

Plato taught that beautiful language could induce *sophrosyne*, a condition of stability and integration in psychic life. Beautiful language was given names by the Greeks of 'epode' and 'theklerian' – charms and spells that could evoke in the listener the experience of calm and well-being.[2] This recognition that something inward exists in human beings that can be touched by means other than something physical (like drugs or surgery) and suggests that that 'within' is important to the process of healing and further, Plato tells us, that this 'within' can be reached through 'beautiful language'.

A leader in the field of medical humanities and a superb poet, Jack Coulehan MD recently wrote me an email, speaking directly to this capacity of poetry to connect with us inwardly. His letter was synchronistic in that he did not know I had just begun my essay by making reference to Plato's 'beautiful language'.

Here Jack responds to my chapter title, 'Healing the within':

> The more I think about this stuff, and the more I teach (using poetry and other creative writing), the more I'm convinced that our goal ought to be to help students become more reflective, more aware of the 'within'; forget the legalistic or intellectual stuff like biomedical ethics, and even forget teaching communication skills as such – only if they can get in touch with themselves will they be willing to listen to others, or respect them.
>
> We often associate the statement 'Know thyself' with Socrates (via Plato), forgetting that 'Know thyself' was the major inscription on the temple of Apollo at Delphi, and that Apollo was the original god of both medicine and poetry – in Apollo the two disciplines seamlessly meld.

Increasingly, a significant number of people in medicine, like Jack Coulehan, recognise poetry's capacity to help us reflect upon life – which also means reflecting on patients, illness, dying, health

'Esparragal, or The Place of Wild Asparagus' by Maxine Relton (original watercolour painting) 'Esparragal' was painted in Andalusia, southern Spain. The door of a cool farmhouse swung open to the light and warmth of day suggests a simple receptivity and natural access I associate with the subject of my chapter: healing, creativity and caring. Tender colours, ripe fruit, streaming light and the human world of a rough-hewn chair are held in place by an invisible generative presence that is, like poetry, capable of opening the heart and reaching us where we live.

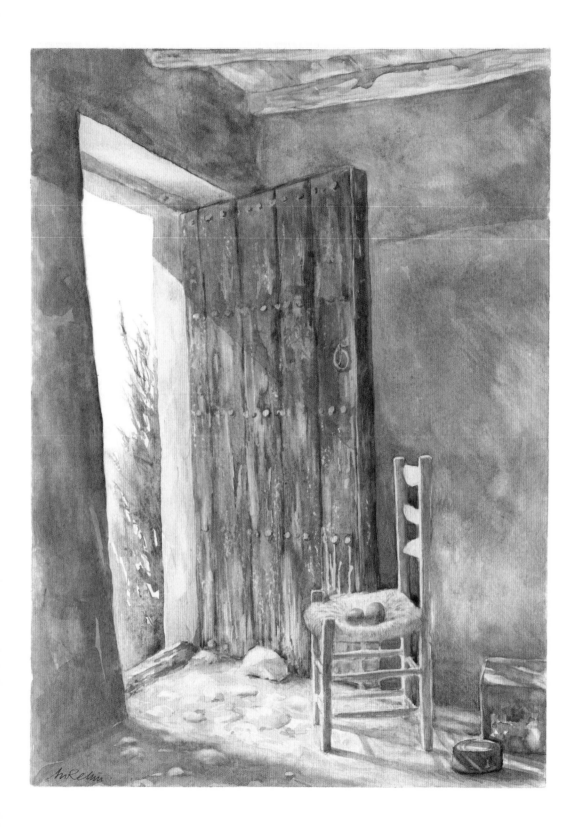

159

and ourselves with more insight and compassion. Poetry therapy is a growing field with certified and registered practitioners at work in hospitals, particularly in America, but the field is also gaining international recognition. Reflective writing and the creation of portfolios by health care professionals, advanced by the work of Gillie Bolton and others, is well rooted in the UK.[3]

Western or allopathic medicine recognises expressive writing, more and more, as a valuable tool. Clinical research shows expressive writing to improve aspects of immune system function and, in studies published by the Journal of the American Medical Association, to ameliorate symptoms of asthma and rheumatoid arthritis.

There is research being done in the UK on the healing potential of writing. Sally Balfe, in an article entitled 'Writing for health' in the online magazine *Positive health*, states that

> Dr Robin Philipp, of Bristol Royal Infirmary conducted research into the health benefits of writing poetry. Of the 200 study participants, 56% said that writing poetry reduced anxiety and provided an emotional outlet. Some said that writing poetry helped them to cope with the pain of bereavement, while others were able to stop taking anti-depressants or tranquillisers.[4]

What ancient cultures once knew about poetry, prayer and chants is coming alive again.

Rafael Campo MD practises at Beth Israel Deaconess Hospital in Boston, Massachusetts, and teaches in the Harvard Medical School. Campo has written widely on poetry and medicine:

> Everything about being human is in poetry, from the rhythms of the heart to the complex responses to fear and desires and pondering our own mortality. Poetry speaks to all of that – and in some ways a lot better than medicine does.[5]

Encouraging changes are happening in medical education and practice, such as the growth of medical humanities and integrative medicine departments. But in general there is a lack of appreciation and attention given to the things to which Coulehan and Campo refer, in both the education and practice of medicine.

Poetry and the healing environment

*The very fact that a thing – anything – can be fitted into a meaning
built up of words, small black words, that can be written with one
hand and the stub of a pencil, means it is not big enough to be
overwhelming. It is the vast, formless, unknown and unknowable
things we fear. Anything which can be brought to a common point –
a focus within our understanding – can be dealt with.*[6]

– Lara Jefferson

Where is the language of poetry found? What creates an optimum
healing environment? Wonder and pain, insight and feeling,
connection and isolation, details and dreams, those things we
know and what we don't, our rich sensing of the natural world and
our intuitive awareness of spirit – this is the stuff of human experience and of poetry. These refer us to our inner world, they reveal
the 'within' of a person. Drawing from a splendidly various range
of sources, poetry can guide us into the wide realms where the
shape of words connects the feeling heart to the world we inhabit.

Mary Oliver shows us this deep sense of 'within' and the way it
joins her to the world in the following poem:

AT BLACKWATER POND

At Blackwater Pond the tossed waters have settled
after a night of rain.
I dip my cupped hands. I drink
a long time. It tastes
like stone, leaves, fire. It falls cold
into my body, waking the bones. I hear them
deep inside me, whispering
oh what is that beautiful thing
that just happened?

Oliver employs her curiosity and senses, her attention to detail
and what is not explainable. Above all, she takes her time and
feels. She cups her hands to receive. She tastes the water and
notices what happens. Read 'At Blackwater Pond' out loud, to your-
self, to a friend. As you read, listen for those places where you
might pause slightly; savour the words and rest in the spaces
between them.

The healing environment flourishes in this way; by taking the same kind of time and offering the same kind of attention. Time and attention establish a safe and sacred place for individuals who are ill and in pain, who face uncertainty, who need to be supported during recovery or in the process of dying. Within that place of safety, trust, empathy, non-judgement, honesty and the capacity to witness are needed. These are the threads of relationship that make an intimately woven fabric of healing and meaningful connection. Such qualities and attitudes *make it possible* to touch another person with comfort, build their faith and even communicate joy. The cultivation of these attitudes within a health care relationship can help people to remember and then rekindle their resilience. They help us to know ourselves and to understand and validate the experience of another person. Employing such attitudes can help to create a place where, as Dr Coulehan says, the disciplines of poetry and medicine 'seamlessly meld'.

Poetry teaches us how to listen deeply, silently. In the process of listening, we come to understand the significance of the words we and others use. Poetry shows us that listening and speaking matter. It provides a container for our perceptions, insights and emotions so that we can first express, and then reflect upon and gradually integrate our experience. Writing transforms, as Lara Jefferson says, the overwhelming, the vast, the formless – into a point within the focus of our understanding.

To listen and speak with intention is to become more present. When we are present in our speaking and listening, we slow down; we can, as Mary Oliver says, 'dip our cupped hands' and in doing that, our senses naturally become more aware of non-verbal cues that speak to us or that we communicate to others. *Presence* is what breathes at the core of the healing environment. Even when a shared language is missing, and perhaps, even more, when there are no words at all, there is still room for connection and presence.

Lianne Mercer RN MSN CPT, a nurse and a poetry therapist, writes of a meeting she had with a patient in her poem 'Bendición':

BENDICIÓN

In Room 28, an old woman perches on her bed
stiff with fear. She licks crooked, gold-filled teeth,
spews Spanish words of sorrow that fall like tears.
I hold out my hands like sieves dripping syllables, say
No comprendo. Ah, she makes the sign of the cross.
Her long fingers reach for mine.

She smiles around my tentative use of *dolor* and *las flores*,
words spoken on this dusky evening eventual night will
    extinguish.
She enriches me – reveals me to myself growing in a dawn
    garden
where zinnias reach for the sun with mariachi arms, where
clicking beetles make music far sweeter than excuses of
    language
blooming, then fading, in our hands.

I breathe in this gift of recognition
from a bent-over woman whose heart bursts
with words needing no voice, spilling
from her eyes into mine, dancing now
beneath our fingers, affirming that we are kin,
breath of feathers on my arm,
whispers in my soul.

Lianne had this to say about writing her poem:

> Writing 'Bendición' was the best way to share my experience,
> to let other people know about the subtle variety of connec-
> tions that are present with another person, even without
> language. What I learned was to not be afraid to give what I
> have – what I am – to give even though I think it might not
> work. It pushed me gently out of my professional comfort
> zone. This patient showed me that I need to risk communi-
> cating in whatever way I can because communication is the
> road into healing.
>
> The second stanza is an affirmation of our common
> humanity. It's about what she gave me. I saw through our
> exchange that it's an accident of circumstance that she is the
> patient and I am the nurse. I saw, through her eyes, that what

she wants is what I want for myself as well – to be understood. In understanding, in that moment of connection, healing can come. Because I can accept whatever is going on with her, I have the chance to accept what is going on inside me. And vice versa. I felt that we both heard and understood each other even without words. It was the touching that made the difference.

In approaching poetry and creative writing in a therapeutic and healing sense, in a way that allows us to explore what matters, I am talking about a way of relating to literature other than what we may have experienced in school. I am not talking about ripping a poem apart as you may have done at school, where you may have dissected to death pieces you had no interest in – or even worse, those you loved! Experiencing poetry from a healing perspective involves trust, empathy, non-judgement and a witnessing presence as a way to learn from another human being – and that's just what I am asking of you as you listen to, learn from and experience a poem.

The poet Donald Hall distils what I mean:

> I would tell him, for instance, that he should not ask for a poem to do any particular thing. I would ask him to relax and listen and float. I would ask him to allow himself to associate. To read a poem you must stop paraphrasing, stop 'thinking' in the conventional way, and do some receiving instead.[7]

Jelaluddin Rumi, a Sufi mystic poet of the twelfth century, encourages a similar approach.

> Listen to the presences inside of poems.
> Let them take you where they will.
>
> Follow those private hints,
> And never leave the premises.

Through getting to know poetry and poetic language in this way, by following where the poem takes you and openly receiving what it means to you *individually*, you will very likely find ways to experience the 'within'.

Starting to write

We may have lost faith in our ability to write poems, just as we have lost faith in our ability to heal. Recovering the poet strengthens the healer and sets free the unique song that is at the heart of every life.

– Dr Rachel Naomi Remen in the preface to *Poetic medicine*[8]

A father once told me, with a deep regret on his face and in his eyes, that he wished his adult daughter would bring him a poem. I asked why. He said that when his daughter was a young girl she brought him one of her poems. He, a sports editor of a city newspaper, was certainly not an insensitive man, but he was an editor, and after all, spelling was important. So, the first thing he said upon reading her poem, as an editor and 'responsible' father, was 'Honey, you've spelled these words wrong…'

She hasn't shared a poem with him since. Now, with appreciation for what really matters, he realises spelling isn't all that important but his daughter and her poems are.

Experiences with our creativity don't always fit into either a positive or negative category. Things don't land just one way or the other. A person has often travelled a more complex journey.

Audrey Shafer is a physician and poet with a lifelong connection with medicine, writing and language.

I was a voracious reader as a child and in second grade I wrote a book of short poems and illustrated them with my set of cray-pas. One of the poems read: 'In the valley of the earth, little women come to work'. I think this was a response to the death of the character Beth in Louisa May Alcott's book *Little women*, which affected me greatly.

Furthermore, my father was a friend of some Philadelphia-area poets, and in particular I recall attending a poetry reading by Gerald Stern at the Painted Bride when I was a little kid. Stern read something about a Fanta orange soda bottle and I remember being incredulous that you could put that sort of thing in a poem. Later, in my high school library I used to listen to recordings of poets and was completely entranced by Dylan Thomas' lush Welsh accent.

About six months after my father's suicide, when I was fifteen years old, I wrote a poem and kept it, for years, in the dust balls under my bed. I'd like to say that it was comforting to have it there, or to have written it, but it wasn't. It was a sore that wouldn't heal properly, and I think that poem became a metaphor, or perhaps merely a poor substitute, for my feelings about the whole thing. And now, on my laptop, I still have an unfinished (or unfinishable!) poem about this loss.

However, it wasn't until medical school and fellowship training that I took some poetry workshops, one with British poet, Denise Levertov, at Stanford. From that point on, writing became part of me – something that I would do erratically, yet somehow the process of writing became a necessity.

The main intersection between my work as an anesthesiologist and my writing is an interest in language. Medicine has its own jargon and terminology, the learning of which is part of the rite of passage to physicianhood. How that language changes when the patient is or is not incorporated into the conversation is fascinating to me. I like paying attention to the language used in the preoperative holding area and when the patient is newly brought into the operating room. Then how the language changes once the patient is anesthetized.

The poem 'One morning' was born of a free write, which is how I frequently 'limber up'. Hence it was a kind of 'bottom up' poem in that I was playing with the word 'lump' and how discrepant the word's implication and its sound were. I chose to reserve the word till the end, to try to mimic the shock of finding a breast lump in a routine morning shower self-exam.

ONE MORNING

a word mocked her
innocently Seussed her
bumpity bumped her
dim light ghostie

the word seemed so plain jane
too slumpy grumpy
for a sloe-eyed morning

how ridiculous – it couldn't be
rumpin' 'n' jumpin'
glee of unleashed dogs

but no – there it was
stump clump

pirates on deck
crimp crump
wrinkle-mouth spinster

sump pump
sewer dump

the river before
the dry creekbed after

one morning
in the shower
fingers stumble

a word forms
its small weight

her tongue whispers

lump

Some words fit their meanings very well – not just onomatopoeic words but also others. Words like 'skunk' or 'thunder'. But the implications of finding a breast 'lump' can be so devastating – not at all captured by the prosaic, playdough sound of the word.

I think, in the practice of medicine, words frequently fail us as well. For instance, there is no good, simple way to describe a general anesthetic to a patient. 'You will be anesthetized' sounds sterile, forbidding and metallic. The word 'sleep' is used to be reassuring, but it is inadequate and inaccurate. Similarly, 'unconscious', 'out', 'under', etc all have problems with them.

Language is fascinating to me – both as a means of, and a barrier to, communication. My poem, 'One morning', is an attempt to contemplate both the inadequacy and the resonance of language. I think my interest in writing has helped me be more keenly aware of how different the patient's perspective is from the health care worker's. Hopefully this interest has improved my sensitivity to the patient's needs, worries and hopes.

Audrey is aware of the limitations and potentials of the large and varied landscapes of both medicine and poetry which for her include both dangerous chasms and verdant walking trails.

Curing anguish, causing joy

Poetry is indeed something divine. It is at once the centre and circumference of knowledge; it is that which comprehends all science, and that to which all science must be referred. It is at the same time the root and blossom of all other systems of thought; it is that from which all spring, and that which adorns all; and that which, if blighted, denies the fruit and the seed, and withholds from the barren world the nourishment and the succession of the scions of the tree of life.[9]

   – Percy Bysshe Shelley

By failing to read or listen to poets, a society dooms itself to inferior modes of articulation – those of the politician, or the salesman or the charlatan… Poetry is not a form of entertainment, and in a certain sense not even a form of art, but our anthropological, genetic goal, our linguistic, evolutionary beacon. We seem to sense this as children, when we absorb and remember verses in order to master language. As adults, however, we abandon this pursuit, convinced that we've mastered it. Yet what we've mastered is but an idiom, good enough perhaps to outfox an enemy, to sell a product, to get laid, to earn a promotion, but certainly not good enough to cure anguish or cause joy.[10]

   – Joseph Brodsky

What Shelley and Brodsky say is not unlike prior comments made by medical practitioners who also happen to write poems – they all recognise poetry as something that is not just valuable for its superb linguistic qualities, but as a biological, ecological and onto-logical reality.

If that is the case, is it not possible that poetry can help us to *know ourselves*?

A contemporary Greek poet and winner of the 1979 Nobel Prize in Literature, the late Odysseus Elytis, shares a story that may help us better appreciate why the inscription 'Know thyself' was written on the healing temple of Apollo and what that has to do with poetry.

Elytis describes the medicinal and protective powers ascribed to sound and language as he recollects the acceptance those 'charms and spells' once enjoyed in his culture, even during his lifetime:

> until a few years ago our island nurses, with utter seriousness, chased evil spirits from above our cradles by uttering words without meaning, holding a tiny leaf of a modest herb which received God knows what strange powers exclusively from the innocence of its own nature.
>
> Poetry is precisely this tiny leaf with the unknown powers of innocence and the strange words which accompany it.[11]

Indeed, the idea that poetry could protect you from illness (ie be a preventative), help you cope with pain and trauma and, even more, regain your balance and wholeness, was once widely accepted as a recognised 'action' of poetic language.[12]

With other cultures, including the enlightened society of India's Vedas, Native American peoples or other indigenous groups, valuing poetic language and the creative imagination is a way to effect healing and serves as a guide for living. In marked contrast, in our modern society, medicine and science seem at odds with poetry. This may be because a poetic sensibility leads us in the direction of the unknown, an area which cannot be scientifically explained, a spiritual realm.

Joseph Bruchac, whose Native American Abenaki ancestry greatly influences his writing, speaks of the place creative language deserves beside other medicinal interventions; how it is intended, in his native understanding of medicine, to establish a more complete relationship with a person who seeks healing:

THE REMEDIES

Half on the Earth, half in the heart,
the remedies for all the things
which grieve us wait for those who know
the words to use to find them.

Penobscott people used to make
a medicine for cancer from Mayapple
and South American people knew
the quinine cure for malaria
a thousand years ago.

But it is not just in the roots,
the stems, the leaves,
the thousand flowers
that healing lies.
Half of it lives within the words
the healer speaks.
And when the final time has come
for one to leave this Earth
there are no cures,
for Death is only
part of Life, not a disease.

Half on the Earth, half in the heart,
the remedies for all our pains
wait for the songs of healing.

Bruchac is aware that his poem about roots, flowers and songs is not aligned with a modern, pharmaceutically 'sophisticated', medical model. His poem purposefully challenges assumptions about modern medical knowledge. He wants to stir our curiosity. The last three lines invite us to consider that our experience of 'the within' in medicine, while seemingly missing, may not in fact be lost. Instead, whatever grieves in us waits to hear 'songs of healing'. People want words that reach their hearts and acknowledge wholeness.

If only our modern day healers knew or could relearn such healing songs. Unfortunately, a practitioner's ability to make use of the evocative nature of poetic language and the skills of reflection to better understand illness and feel empathy for patients has not *only* been abandoned. It has also been supplanted by technical jargon, accounting concerns, marketing and specialisation. Metaphor, mystery and a heart-connection between caregiver and patient have lost their natural places in our lives.

Does this loss of spiritual connection within the modern medical community stem from our overdependence on what we can prove as fact? The absence of heart-connection, which poetry so naturally fosters, is not just a health care system dilemma; it's a human one.

One of the UK's foremost poets, Dannie Abse, a retired physician, uses imagination, compassion and irony to show us some of the consequences of practising medicine in a way disconnected from life and mystery.

LUNCH WITH A PATHOLOGIST

My colleague knows by heart the morbid verse
of facts – the dead weight of a man's liver,
a woman's lungs, a baby's kidneys.

At lunch he recited unforgettably,
'After death, of all soft tissue the brain's
the first to vanish, the uterus the last.'

'Yes,' I said, 'at dawn I've seen silhouettes
hunched in a field against the skyline, each one
feasting, preoccupied, silent as gas.

'Partial to women, they've stripped woman bare
and left behind only the taboo food,
the uterus, inside the skeleton.'

My colleague wiped his mouth with a napkin,
hummed, picked shredded meat from his canines,
said, 'You're a peculiar fellow, Abse.'

– Dannie Abse

Naturally, both patients and physicians seek 'cures' and 'facts'. We rightly want solutions that work and make us better. Yet, something is lost from this process if we don't consider the underlying causes of illness, when we carry on in our busy lives without making essential changes or recognising the opportunity for what John Keats called 'soul-making'. Whether patients are ultimately torn apart by illness, die or get better, they will need the support of the medical establishment as they explore their living and reflect upon their eventual dying. Without that connection, without support for reflection and learning, their experience of health care delivery may become distanced, uncompassionate and fragmented.

Patient and physician need a language that describes this journey of illness, dying and of getting well again, a journey which so often does not offer neatly packaged answers, but may pose questions, suggest choices, require time, evoke feeling and leave paradoxes.

They also require a language that helps physician and patient celebrate progress and cope with and learn from uncertainty and loss.

Poetry offers this potent, distilled language. A poem gets to the heart of things. It is a natural medicine that extends solace and relief, gives a cathartic voice to suffering, reveals insight and shows us what it means to be human. Dr Charles Perakis' poem, 'Mary Rivers', offers such medicine and reveals the need for a way to listen that increases empathy and establishes connection:

MARY RIVERS

Mary was my patient for less than four months.
Ovarian cancer can be ugly.
Hers was.
When I first met her
she weighed only 86 pounds.
Chemotherapy had not helped
and took her hair.
Her belly was distended
with fluid.
Talk of her illness or family
produced rapid bursts of tears.
She rewarded my care
and presence
with a lesson in dying.
I pronounced her dead
at her home.
I took the long way
back to my office
to let my tears dry.

Charles Perakis is an osteopathic family physician and medical school teacher who has spent much of his professional life exploring connections between medicine and the arts. This is what he had to say about his writing, his practice of medicine, and the need for physicians to reflect on and listen to the human beings they are treating:

Mary Rivers is from a series I wrote about people, my patients; poems reminiscent of Edgar Lee Masters' *Spoon River anthology.*

I have apple crates in my cellar full of patients' charts. I picked out the dying patients' charts, people who made a particularly powerful emotional impact on me. I took my clinical problem-oriented soap notes, which were written in a medical tone. They are not poetic. Upon reflection, I wrote the poems. I wanted to be more personal, to reflect on my vulnerability and also capture the essence of that person and my experience in a poem. When I went back, looking behind my clinical notations, I realized I was going through the process of confronting mortality.

I hadn't taken care of a lot of dying patients at that time. There wasn't much I could do for Mary other than be there for her. That was the biggest lesson I learned: that I didn't have to do anything except be present and listen. Sometimes it's much easier for a doctor to do something. Mary taught me about being present, even with my discomfort. I knew she was going to die and it was tough.

Writing these poems about patients influences my teaching now. I believe that practice is research and I am always trying to figure out how I can do practice better. Physicians are always trying to figure out what practice is so we need to reflect on what we did today. Emphasis on the science part of medicine has taken us away from that reflection. We need a method to remind us to reflect.

The method that I've found that really works is the portfolio and that often includes poetry. A lot of my students write poetry, sometimes at my suggestion and sometimes on their own. Poetry is a language of reflection. I see reflection as an essential element to making a humane physician and to the development of an empathetic practice.

When you are a generalist you realise that a lot of the things people present are based on predicaments, they are not because of disease. Someone got fired, there is not enough money, there is domestic violence, or drug abuse. It's not what you usually find in an internal medicine textbook. Predicaments are much more complex. It takes a lot of reflection to figure out what's going on. The treatment for that person and their predicament is not writing a prescription, the treatment is often being present and listening. That's what the person needs. That practice of listening is devalued. The specialist may think it's an easy thing to do, but it's not an easy thing to do.

The soulful story of human struggle in the midst of illness and death, the will to persevere and heal and thrive, letting go of what was to accept what is – poetry expresses these authentically, with an immediacy and impact that clinical language cannot achieve.

Summary

As a poetry therapist I am interested in exploring the uses of writing and speaking poems to:

> ▷ increase self-awareness and self-care;
> ▷ support the release of hurt and pain;
> ▷ help a person make healthy connections with self and others; and,
> ▷ open up a consideration of a spiritual dimension to life.

When we listen to or read poetry, when we respond to or write it, there is a chance to slow down and notice our lives. We reflect on what's written on the page in order to integrate what's living in the heart.

We pour into the healing environment of the blank page, this sacred container: letters, words, pauses, rhythms and sounds of 'just this much' of our lives.

That is, we give voice to what's true for us right now: an experience we disclose, an insight we discover, a wound we disinfect, a hurt we name and so begin to disentangle ourselves from.

The poetry therapist is trained to help a person or a group of people work with their writing so that it can serve them in their search for meaning. We believe that poetry provides us with another way to relate to the complexity of illness, suffering and our will towards well-being.

Healing poetry offers a nurturing and more sustainable environment than the thin, poor soil which comprises the vast grey agribusiness that defines much of modern life, including exclusive reliance on a biomedical model of disease that fails to recognise the wholeness and mystery of a human being.

Poetic language, rich with metaphor, image and symbol, makes it possible for us to express the diverse, paradoxical, vibrant organisms we are – human beings that grow and struggle, sometimes get ill and heal, live and die, sorrow and sing.

Because poetry puts words together in imaginative ways, not the exacting ways of a grammarian, it allows individuals to explore their lives in ways that can be surprising.

The magic of words offers a person a pathway to enter a new and creative viewpoint. It opens us up to a channel of insight, to something we don't know rationally but something we inherently recognise, feel and understand.

To a person dealing with illness, to a physician attending to that patient, to apprehend this moment of recognition on the part of the patient can initiate an empathic resonance between patient and physician, foster a healing environment and make all the difference in their relationship.

The poet Adrienne Rich observes 'the moment of change is the only poem'. How do we note such change as poetry therapists? When people are moved by a poem they write or hear spoken, there is often a sigh, a deep nod of the head; the person may sit up straighter, and the comment is often made aloud by those listening to the person, 'Read it again!'

If we can enter that moment of change with someone, enter it with our deep listening and attention, people say that such a simple, direct act is a gift. They say deep listening holds, witnesses, validates, roots, affirms, connects, respects, is generative. When illness impacts our lives these positive effects of listening are especially needed, helpful and treasured. This experience can show us in a helping profession what it means to be a healer. It can show someone who is ill, who feels broken and scared, what it means to be loved and to come home to oneself.

But it is not enough to tell you this. There is an old aphorism about writing poetry that says, 'Show, don't tell'. So I will.

When I began my internship to become a poetry therapist in 1985 it suddenly became clear to me that it was in this kind of listening that I had the most to learn from and through which I could also help the most. It was during this time the following poem 'arrived'.

WHEN SOMEONE LISTENS TO YOU

When someone deeply listens to you
it is like holding out a dented cup
you've had since childhood

and watching it fill up with
cold, fresh water.
When it balances on top of the brim,
you are understood.
When it overflows and touches your skin,
you are loved.

When someone deeply listens to you
the room where you stay
starts a new life
and the place where you wrote
your first poem
begins to glow in your mind's eye.
It is as if gold has been discovered!

When someone deeply listens to you
your bare feet are on the earth
and a beloved land that seemed distant
is now at home within you.

– John Fox

Note

For more information about poetry therapy, contact the National Association for Poetry Therapy, 16861 SW 6th Street, Pembroke Pines, FL 33027, USA. Email **NAPTstarr@aol.com** or visit the website at **www.poetrytherapy.org**

References

1 Greifer E. *Principles of poetry therapy.* New York: Poetry Therapy Centre, 1963.
2 Morrison MR. The use of poetry in the treatment of emotional dysfunction. *The Arts in Psychotherapy*, 5:93–98.
3 Bolton G. *Reflective practice: writing and professional development.* London: Paul Chapman Publishing Ltd, 2001.
4 Balfe S, 'Writing for health', www.positivehealth.com/permit/Articles/Stress/Balfe33.html
5 Quoted in: Shelton DL, 'Healing words', *American Medical News*, 17 May 1999.
6 Jefferson L. *These are my sisters.* New York: Double-Day Book Company, 1952.
7 Hall D. Source unknown.

8   Fox J. *Poetic medicine: the healing art of poem-making.* New York: Tarcher/Putnam, 1997.

9   Shelley PB. *A defence of poetry.* 1821, 1840.

10 Brodsky J, 'An immodest proposal', an address delivered at the Library of Congress, Washington DC, October 1991.

11 Elytis O. *Open paper: selected essays.* Port Townsend, WA: Copper Canyon Press, 1995.

12 Joy Shieman was influential in helping me to formulate this idea.

12

The medical paradigm: changing landscapes

ROGER HIGGS

Professor Roger Higgs, general practitioner and medical ethicist, reflects on the changing relationship between doctors and patients, and the several needs and aspirations these changes represent. He argues that changing relations reflect and inform wider societal ideas about the nature of medicine and of society in our time.

Waking up after the tonsil operation, I lay on a rubber sheet that smelt like the gas mask I had played with at the back of our attic. The metal window of the hut came and went in the late afternoon sunshine. An Essex voice, somewhere out there, said, 'No, his mother can come tomorrow'. I cried myself into sleep, and woke at night to the sound of men's laughter and burping. The smell of cigarette smoke added to the taste of blood. I was in hospital, in the men's ward. It was 1949. I was very big – nearly six.

Fifty years on, after a working life as both hospital doctor and GP, and involvement in the medical system as a patient and a relative of patients, I see a very different picture of health care in the UK. For all of us the landscape we live in changes so gradually, so relentlessly, that we often do not remember what it used to be like. In this century, in the UK, it would probably be a matter of complaint if a mother could not see her five-year-old very soon after an operation. If she found him in a bed beside adult men, there would be headlines in *The Sun* newspaper and an enquiry. I can't swear the smoking was actually in the ward: after all, it was a big Nissen hut-type room and the outside world with grass and trees was just beyond the black rubber swing doors. Nowadays, if you smell cigarette smoke as a patient in a hospital you've probably strayed into the resident staff sitting room or managed to get all the way down to the hospital exit. Hospitals nowadays are usually huge and often beautiful buildings, with even the children's wards remote from grass or trees.

 If the buildings are different, the way we use them, and what is achieved within them, has also altered, in some cases beyond recognition. A child of six just diagnosed with a potentially lethal leukaemia will probably be *cured* in the dawning biotechnological revolution. Her parents will probably be able to see her as often as they like, perhaps even by staying on the ward. The fear of not getting out of hospital – a common fear in the 1940s – has been replaced by concern about the difficulty of getting seen as quickly as you would want to, and of getting *into* hospital when necessary; postponed outpatients appointments, cancelled admissions and long delays to reach the head of the investigation queue are all like a sickening hangover from the heady advances and underinvestment in health care that have characterised the last fifty years. But the perceived problems with today's health care system do not just revolve around resources. Modern views of benefit and risk for children mean that persuading someone to remove your child's tonsils requires dedication and persistence of a high order. If you do manage that task then, the cynic might say, you will need more of the same to find the doctor, and perhaps more again to find a language you can both use freely in order to make progress.

 But while the landscape of health care that patients and professionals live in has changed, so, it seems, has the landscape that lives within the patients and professionals. If medicine thinks differently about patients – on subjects as diverse as the benefits to a child of keeping his tonsils to the personal and social costs of a long stay in hospital – so society has changed the way it thinks about medicine. I will argue that half a century ago, when attempting suicide was a crime and being gay was a disease,* suffering was different, and best done quietly and alone. Ironically, given what we now know about the adverse health effects of smoking tobacco, in the 1940s smoking was actively encouraged as a way of coping with life and the challenges it offered. In 1952,

---

*Attempted suicide was decriminalised in England and Wales in 1961; in the following decade psychiatrists were still treating people for homosexuality (which was also still a crime).

when the monarch, King George VI, died of lung cancer, there was no outcry about the disease or its obvious cause. The King was respected, as I remember, for his quiet determination and for getting on with the job like everyone else. Doctors too were there just to do their job. Being humane was not part of what was expected of them.

The picture that I saw from my bed in the Nissen hut back in 1949 was not what I would see now. The physical landscape of medicine has changed, and the scope and style of medical practice with it. But more interesting to me, as an observer both inside and outside the medical care system in UK, is the emotional and moral landscape; what has altered in the human, internal territory of behaviour and attitudes, in people's values and how they like to express them. I would like to explore how these are revealed when people are ill, or think they may be, and come to get professional help. I would also like to reflect on how I have seen that emotional and moral landscape change, and then look at what it means to *suffer* in the early twenty-first century. It will be a brief and personal study which looks at some interactions between people and their chosen clinicians to try to understand the terms in which these discussions are framed. It is my view that there is a new way of suffering which is also reshaping the framework within which medical practice is conducted, and changing, perhaps, its very paradigm.

This will be an account which largely depends on my own observations, as a student, hospital doctor, general practitioner, and teacher in medical ethics and primary care. But as well as looking at meetings between patients and clinicians, the ideas are also refracted through encounters between people and special buildings or paintings. There is a long tradition in Western thinking which avers that the handling of moral values and attitudes in human nature is closely linked to our aesthetic judgements. Shaftesbury, and later Hume, saw that the 'moral sense is like the sense of beauty in that it detects the "moral beauty" that is present in the ways that persons respond to other persons'.[1] Modern psychological thinking sees similar links between moral and aesthetic choices.[2] This connection can both clarify and confuse, but whether it helps or hinders, it certainly exists. It helps by holding up a mirror to human nature through art. It helps to explain why the careful design of new environments is so important. It helps to show why 'the humanities', as they are currently referred to in the academic world, may have something important to say about humane behaviour in medical care.

The importance of relationships in medicine

Although the scope and techniques of medicine have changed, the relationships we all make and experience as we deliver or receive medical care continue to matter. So I shall begin by looking at the relationship between two individuals; a person with a problem and a person paid to provide a response. But the question asked by patients, 'What is happening to me?' brings with it another question: 'What is the me it is happening to?' and so I will also focus on a less examined relationship; that between the two individuals meeting and their own inner selves.

I will begin this analysis by outlining the factors that I believe have, during my professional lifetime, been influential in the changing nature of the doctor–patient relationship from a paternalistic to a partnership-based one. I will also map out my understanding of the evolving nature of understanding that individuals within our society have of their inner selves, as well as advances in medical appreciation of the role that the relationship between the doctor's and the patient's inner selves have on the quality of the medical encounter. I will suggest that if the importance of this relationship, between the inner selves of a person with a problem and a person paid to provide a response, is not properly acknowledged and understood then this can act as a barrier to the formation of a good doctor–patient partnership.

From paternalism to partnership: the changing doctor–patient relationship

In 1949, the doctor–patient relationship was a paternalistic one. The response to emergencies and extreme time pressure was clear and workmanlike. The doctor's questions were focused on the matter in hand; irrelevant issues were excluded. During an era immediately after the war when people still tended to obey orders, this process at least had the merit of having outcomes and using the time appropriately. The doctor made the diagnosis; the patient was told what should be done. The patient's or relative's aims and views did not usually enter the frame. The new NHS, born just before that year when I was in the Nissen hut,* may have altered the background of encounters between doctors and patients, but the details of what actually occurred within the doctor–patient encounter took far longer to change.

As late as the 1960s, the session advertised as ethics teaching for my class of medical students in London was still only about the 'rule of As' – no abortion, adultery, alcoholism, advertising or associations with unlicensed practitioners of any kind.[3] The focus was on traditional rules, which were largely concerned with medical values, not with the values held by patients. No challenges were made to the concept that doctors always knew what was best for their patients, and should therefore decide what should be done. When, two years later, I suggested a discussion of more modern, less paternalistic, approaches at the hospital where I was training, a consultant neurologist joked, 'Higgs, when I hear the word "ethics" I reach for my golf clubs'.† There was for him no point in discussing medical paternalism because it was how he worked, and for him it worked well.

Wider social changes and their impact on medicine

While the changes inside medicine were slow in coming, those occurring outside medicine were rapid and far-reaching. For my older companions in the Nissen hut in the 1940s it had been glorious just to be 'young, alive and unwounded',[4] but the 1950s demanded more. 'You've never had it so good,' said Prime Minister Harold MacMillan in 1957, to which our generation joked in reply (with some truth) that we'd never had it.‡ By the 1960s, relationships in general were under the microscope. The Quaker pamphlets

---

*The British NHS, planned during the Second World War and introduced by Attlee's Labour Government, became law in 1946 but was not effective until 1948. It set up a comprehensive health service paid for by the state, offering free diagnosis and treatment at home or in hospital to every person in the country.

†He was a cultured man and enjoyed teasing, and knew I should be riled by the echoes of 'Whenever I hear the word culture, I reach for my pistol', attributed to the Nazi Hermann Goering.

‡Harold MacMillan said this from a speech at Bedford on 20 July 1957, echoing a slogan in a recent US election.

about same-sex relationships,[5] the 'Honest to God' debate,[6] and the forward thinking by John Bowlby on attachment in childhood,[7] were all, in hindsight, indications of a new democracy, beyond formal politics, in daily living.

The whole idea that our private lives and our personal behaviour, and so the decisions about our person, were *entirely* our own to decide was at last taking root, tapping into strong subterranean layers of thinking and culture in the West. But the personal consequences of this thinking for all citizens (once votes for women had confirmed that we were all citizens)* must, I suspect, have been held back by the centralising tendencies of two terrible world wars. In the 1960s there was a cheque waiting to be cashed, in medicine as elsewhere. Decisions by an individual about that individual were, at least in principle, to be respected. The era of respect for personal autonomy had at last arrived.

Medical ethics and a quiet revolution

Even if for some this was, and perhaps still is, a false dawn,† the student classes of the 1960s, of which I was a member, were conscious of the illumination of this idea even in the dark recesses of medical education. In the middle of the decade undergraduate medical ethics groups appeared in almost all medical schools in London. Stimulated by the ideas of a progressive Anglican priest, Edward Shotter who worked in London University, discussions began to be held about issues which would now be recognised as core to a twenty-first century curriculum in medical ethics and law. These discussions spread rapidly to most, if not all, medical schools throughout the UK.

The local leadership of these discussion groups was from students, and the style was that of symposia, open to all. Sympathetic senior clinicians would discuss and dispute, and students would challenge and debate. It is probable that for many students

---

*British women over the age of 30 were given the vote in Great Britain in 1918, but women aged between 21 and 30 not until 1928. Women in New Zealand have been able to vote since 1893.

†Examples are limitless but could include the extraordinary way in which women were not allowed into the professions in Britain: the first woman High Court Judge was appointed in 1965. By 1970, still only a quarter of practising doctors in UK were female (and only 6% in the USA).

the excitement lay more in the shifting boundaries of medical care than in moving the borders of personal responsibility: 'Who gets the kidney?' may have been more of a draw than 'Who decides for the individual?' But these arenas of ethical exploration were, nevertheless, significant in moving forward the debate about paternalism and autonomy in medical care.

Not everyone was on board: professional conservatism was strong. One specialist rounded on Shotter, refusing to join a discussion on a medical dilemma by saying, 'These sort of issues should (only) be discussed by consultants, with consultants, and *in camera*'. But the movement was unstoppable. As one of the annual student presidents of the London Medical Group, I was invited by Ted Shotter to join the newly formed Institute of Medical Ethics, which later started what was then (and still is) one of the leading international journals in medical ethics.* While other European students in 1968 were building barricades and uprooting cobble stones, our revolution was quieter and closer to home.

Community health councils and the Lambeth Community Care Centre

When I became a junior doctor I was able to continue working in this new field, and started to provide the editor of the new journal, Alistair Campbell, with discussion about real cases. Some of these provided the background for academic law professor Ian Kennedy's ground-breaking late night TV series on medical ethics.† The debate had now shifted from professional chambers to the public arena. But by then my personal focus had shifted too.

Putting into practice these new views of personal autonomy in medical care was easier in the relative freedom of general practice than in the confines of a hospital ward. I was fortunate, as a young GP in the mid-1970s in South London, to discover two new forces. Community heath councils (CHCs) had been set up to ensure that the patient's voice was properly heard. In Lambeth an inspiring CHC leader, Sue Thorne, was making that a reality by discovering

---

*The *Journal of Medical Ethics* was first published in 1975. It is now part of the BMJ stable, and published jointly with the Institute of Medical Ethics.
†Ian Kennedy had given the 1981 Reith Lectures published subsequently in *The Listener* under the title 'Unmasking medicine'.

what local people wanted from their health care providers. The second force for change was that of more democratic direction within the NHS bureaucracy itself, which acknowledged the contributions and concerns of the community as well as those of hospital management. In the area served by St Thomas's Hospital in London, consulting and supporting the community became something which the local NHS agreed to do. As a consequence, hospitals could not be closed without CHC approval, and new health care developments had to involve the community.

When Lambeth Hospital was threatened with closure in 1976, the CHC brought together a group of local activists and 12 local general practitioners (GPs), including myself. We made it clear that we would agree to this closure only if another facility was provided. This facility would need to bridge the yawning gap between what ill people needed and what could be provided by the NHS locally once the Lambeth Hospital closed. An intermediate facility was required that would look after people when they were too ill to look after themselves, and provided their care was still within the capacity of general practice. It would provide the new skills of terminal care. It would take seriously the care of the chronically ill, particularly in terms of preventing further deterioration by providing physical therapy, rather than just aiming for cure and then abandoning all care if cure could not be achieved. It would provide regular respite relief for carers of disabled people.[8]

Building a local health care setting that empowered individuals

It is strange to record that the battles to set up this new community care facility were long and bitter. The development was opposed by many senior figures in local secondary care and even by some local GPs. Senior echelons of the regional NHS found the concept of an inpatient facility run by general practitioners hard to accept, since it made permeable a division of the NHS which had been key at its birth; that only consultants (and not GPs) should care for those sick enough to need to be in beds. One consultant asked me, 'But can GPs look after people who are *really* ill?'

Both the larger local political parties, apparently wedded to centralising tendencies, rejected the concept of institutional care in the community: the local Labour party at the time saw hospitals as the arbiters of health care. One of the most valuable groups to help us in our thinking was the team of architects involved in the project. Although the planning committee was blocked for some time by the regional NHS from bringing in architects, it was eventually able to appoint the Edward Cullinan Partnership. The architects gave much more time than is usual to helping to get the brief exactly as was needed, both in terms of design and function, and were just as skilled in helping the planning group to progress the project as in creating a beautiful building.[9]

One of the key founding principles of the Lambeth Community Care Centre (LCCC) was that patients were the people who should decide the style of their care. Patients should have their own medicines beside their beds, and should, wherever possible, decide the shape of their lives when they were living there. Patients should have complete access to their medical records, and treatment plans should be discussed and agreed before admission. We in the planning team were looking for a real and realised partnership between an individual and his or her nurse, therapist and doctor which would underline the concept of respecting the autonomy of everyone involved.

Some of the design was created to reflect these driving principles and remind all users of these ideas. Ted Cullinan, the senior member of the team of architects, pointed out that people he knew went upstairs to bed if they lived on two floors, and so he suggested that, in keeping with the way in which people live their lives when not ill, the day centre activity should be on the ground floor and the rooms for patients overnight use upstairs. The front door was secured by a bell and buzzer like a house front door, not by a receptionist. The garden was almost as important as the building, and ten times as disruptive to plan: everyone had their own perfect idea of what a garden (and a therapeutic one at that) should really be like!

In 1985, at long last, the Lambeth Community Care Centre, the first of the new intermediate care centres, was opened. It was planned not as an extension of hospitals out into the community, but as an extension of home care. Wherever possible, individual patients would be helped to carry on with their lives in the routines that they usually used, even though resource constraints and the need for clinical care meant that they had to be in the Centre. To open it, Prince Charles would bring his new wife Diana.

Diana and the common touch

We did not have any inkling then what a potent reminder of patient power and changing times the opening of the Centre by Diana would be. The accompanying media, and through them members of the public throughout the UK, observed with interest the way that Charles and Diana stopped to speak to every patient (and made themselves very late); and that Diana never addressed any of the patients in wheelchairs or beds without going down to their eye level. This in itself was new enough to observers at the time, but when later (and elsewhere) Diana publicly shook hands with a patient with the new and frightening disease of AIDS, those of us working in the Centre realised that an important change was taking place in the power balance within medical care.

AIDS, a totally new disease at that time, was in the popular mind wildly contagious, completely untreatable and a symbol of pollution to the homophobic because of its association with the gay community. Its appearance threatened to push away so much that had been gained in the previous quarter century, and return popular thinking about contamination and diversity back to the Middle Ages. In 1986, the first patient in my general practice to be diagnosed with AIDS was received calmly and courteously into the Lambeth Community Care Centre by staff and fellow patients, and lived his last weeks there with dignity and, importantly for him and for those caring for him, in a style that he was used to. In small but vital ways, the partnership between patients and health care professionals seemed to be taking shape.

A partnership, however, is not necessarily one of equals, nor would it be the model that everyone, even now, would think desirable for a relationship between clinician and patient. In the 1980s, however, it seemed the basic geometry from which more could be developed. One of the GP members of the LCCC planning team, David Poole, described 'the excitement of empowering an individual' – by which he meant patient users of the Centre, though the move towards a doctor–patient partnership could equally well have been argued to offer the possibility of empowerment to professional users.

Critics of these moves might easily say that to *give* real power to patients, it must be *taken* from professionals. But a less powerful professional may not be what would be most helpful to a patient, and some of this debate diverts attention from the real sources of disempowerment for most patients. It is the illness that is really reducing a patient's abilities, even if, in the response to that illness, professional paternalism in some shape or form may come as double jeopardy.

The individual and the inner self

People who are ill resort to professional help for a number of reasons; but one reason, clearly visible in every general practice surgery, is that many people, including professionals, simply do not know enough about themselves to respond appropriately and put things right when they are feeling unwell. To do this may be impossible, like pulling oneself up by one's own shoelaces; but in many cases it is clear to any observer that the person feels ill, or is disturbed by a bodily or mental 'symptom', because they *do not understand themselves*.

An ill person may not understand enough about their basic human nature, make-up, physiology – what you will – but they also often do not know how to reflect on what their desires, disappointments, delinquencies or distress are doing to alter their sense of being well. Some unusual illness behaviour is passed on through families or cultural groups, but it is likely that all people are built on basically similar lines. It is as if human hardware is the same, but the software inserted into each of us is very different.*

So we come to consideration of the second of the two relationships, the relationship between the person and their own inner self. As I said earlier, underlying the apparently straightforward question patients ask within the person-professional partnership, 'What is wrong with me?', lies the more elusive enquiry 'What is the me it is wrong with?' Could it be that most people are like a stranger to their own inner selves; that they sit as uneasily with their own inner lives as they sometimes do with other people? Could it be, in the formulation of 1960s liberation theology, that to live with (and perhaps love) other people we all first have to learn to live with (and love) ourselves?

---

*For an explanation of this image, see Steven Pinker.[2]

The historical landscape of privacy

With the cameras and microphones of the *Big brother* television series intruding into almost every aspect of an individual's life, it is hard to remember how new a phenomenon this opencast mining of the landscape of privacy is. To preserve the private domain, European law has had to reinforce the boundaries between public and private by statute.* Keeping patients' secrets has always been a concern of medical teachers, from the writer or writers of the Hippocratic corpus onwards.

A professional in health care is let in on all sorts of secrets. When I started working in general practice in 1975 and took over a single-handed practice, home visiting was frequently done. I got to know the patients on my list very well. In spite of this, they often presented to me in ways which gave no acknowledgement of this intimacy. It was not at all unusual for people to present pains in tummy, head or back, weight loss or palpitations as diseases in themselves requiring immediate treatment, and not as illnesses perhaps relating in some way to that individual's environment or emotional life. For the doctor to question whether some emotional disturbance or life event might be connected to these symptoms was to risk disrupting the positive flow of the consultation: 'Don't you think I'm ill then?', 'Are you telling me I'm a liar?'

There are several possible interpretations of these responses from patients which were, with notable exceptions, common. As a result of writing about some of these issues in the *British Medical Journal*,[10] a national organisation offered the services of a counsellor to my practice. The excellent professional who came was, unfortunately, not able to generate any insight or reflection within the group of clients or patients whom she saw, and the project was (initially) a failure.† Was the negative response from my patients to the suggestion of psychological worries, and the resistance to the help offered by the counsellor, a hangover from that post-war environment in Britain, where the upper lip was to be kept stiff as much

---

*This was enshrined in Article 8 of the European Convention of Human Rights, and passed as the Human Rights Act 1998.

†After that a colleague, Annalee Curran, developed a new eclectic approach out of antenatal counselling based on cognitive-analytic therapy and responding actively to clients at the level and in the style they found acceptable.[11]

by denial as by bravery? The latter was certainly an interpretation offered to me by overseas colleagues at the time.

Was the problem perhaps a lack of trust or of vocabulary? The concept of somatisation – whereby unacknowledged psychological stresses are manifested as bodily symptoms – is now well established.[12] But that concept only partially covers the phenomenon I was observing then. Whatever the explanation, it is often too painful or too difficult for people to look deeply into their inner selves or the workings of their immediate social group. In one form of family therapy, the unacknowledged feeling within a family is likened to a disaffected soldier, who wages a private guerrilla war on the more conscious rational self of one member of the family, and so on the overt values of the entire family group.[13] It seems possible to me that such a phenomenon could occur within an individual who is not aware of his or her own needs or responses. A minor physical feeling may become the focus, or even the vehicle, of frustrated expression within that individual. Misunderstood pain or other malfunction drives the person to seek help.[14,15]

Helping doctors gain insight into their inner selves

When a patient seeks help from a doctor the response the professional offers might not be what the patient expected. If no disease or physical cause is found, the patient may, as the doctor sees it, have been reassured, but sometimes, frustratingly for doctor and patient, the patient does not feel reassured, and the symptom persists. The patient keeps on coming back. When this happens repeatedly, the first partnership, that between patient and professional, may be sabotaged and something worse, like conflict or rejection, emerges.

The influential psychoanalyst Michael Balint began his important work about these issues[16] by bringing together GPs to talk about patients they really couldn't stand – a group which was later, in more reactionary times, labelled as 'heartsink patients'.[17] But what Balint's groups, under his guidance, came to see was that a 'difficult patient' was caused by a 'difficult doctor'. The professional, with possibly as little insight as the patient, was being approached at one of his or her own special weak spots. It was the interaction of two sinking hearts that created the problem. Groups of GPs, meeting to discuss these issues and make progress in patient care, became important in London, then in the UK, then internationally. Almost all GPs in training now undergo a similar process involving reflection and support.

I have attended such a group with colleagues for all my working life as a GP. The group meets, on average, monthly to examine the interface between professional and personal life. Within the consultation itself, however, something also has to be done if progress is to be made. A technique suggested by Balint's original work was for doctor and patient to set aside a lot more time to understand each other. But that was and remains hard to fit into an already busy routine. A concept that later emerged from Balint groups was that of the sudden intuition (called a 'flash') which might inform the professional: an insight into inner selves, a way of seeing what was going on, a different understanding.

This 'flash' is also reported by professional job interviewers, who describe being very clear in the first moments of some interviews whether a candidate is suitable or not. It seems very similar to the insight of an artist. Such an insight is sometimes something that makes art valuable for others: the artist has in some way 'communicated' her vision. Clearly this is often seen as entirely subjective and a personal experience only. It is a matter of interpretation and there are many possible: most readers will be familiar with the debate. As an interpretation it will not usually lead to action. But intuition is, in human experience, still a powerful and important mechanism which helps us to gain understanding, and so to live with others, and with ourselves. A personal example from outside medicine may be helpful in illustrating this point. It may also suggest other ways in which the humanities remain important to medical practice.

A personal insight from the work of artist Pierre Bonnard

In 1998, the Tate gallery in London put on a major retrospective on the painting of Pierre Bonnard. I knew Bonnard's work reasonably well and was excited by it. He was born in 1867 in Paris, and had an active artist's life till he died in 1947. He is a major colourist, painting ordinary life, particularly interiors, in a way which totally alters one's way of looking at the world. His big oils of the nude in the bath have become modern icons. In his personal life he was a

'The open window' by Pierre Bonnard (1921)

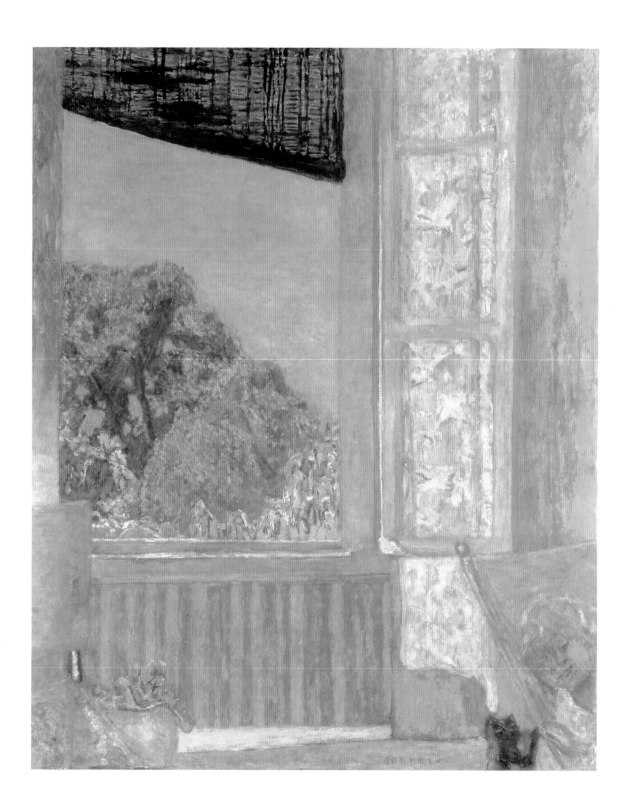

very shy, retiring, intensely private man. He came from a close middle class family, but spent most of his life living with a woman he called Marthe. They met on the street in 1893 when they were both in their twenties. Marthe was not her real name, but she chose to keep her origins a secret for much of their lives together.

Marthe became Bonnard's model and muse: he painted her nearly 400 times, and her rounded face, slim hips and long legs become familiar to anyone looking at Bonnard's work. She too was famously secretive, even reclusive. Although Bonnard's family were apparently welcoming, they knew little about her. She seldom went out alone, and spent much of the latter part of her life bathing and washing, often at spas or in the bath at home. It is not clear whether she had a serious physical condition, for which this was a treatment, or whether she was psychologically unwell. Bonnard's personal life revolved around her, and around caring for her, as well as painting her portrait, slowly and carefully, again and again.

This much I knew when I went to the exhibition, and stopped in front of a painting called *The open window*, which Bonnard had painted in his mid-fifties in 1921. The sight of the painting gripped me suddenly and in a way I could not explain. The picture is of a window opening from the artist's home onto a view of summer trees beyond. The trees are painted in some detail. What is inside the room is less in focus, although the colours are brilliant. To the right we see Marthe, the artist's long-term partner, and her black cat. Across the top of the window is a partly unrolled blind. I had no idea what had arrested me about this particular painting, amongst so many striking images painted by Bonnard and exhibited there together at the Tate, until I began to look more carefully.

The first clue to my reaction was the blind across the top of the window. Instead of being almost straight, as the perspective might suggest, its lower edge was at an angle: hanging between the hot inner room and the cooler world outside it, seemed to me to be like a guillotine blade. I stepped back to look at the catalogue and to read.[18] At the point where the painting was described, there were also shown pages from Bonnard's sketch-book. In one sketch the blind is very obviously skewed, or unevenly unrolled. There is also another sketch, of the trees for the middle of the oil painting. In the sketched trees is a woman's face. But it is not Marthe. It is that of a much younger woman called Renée Monchaty.

Most artists paint from more than one model, and Bonnard was no exception. Renée was one of the models he used. Renée had got to know Bonnard and Marthe when they were both approaching fifty, and Renée was in her twenties. She was a regular visitor at their home and wrote to them both. Bonnard used her as a model quite often, and a painting from 1923 – *Young women in the garden* – shows her surrounded by a halo of yellow.[18] Bonnard kept this painting with him, and in his own possession, till he died.

In 1921, Bonnard and Renée had spent some time together in Rome (the year of the painting of *The open window*), and became lovers. She apparently became his fiancée.[18] In 1924 she went on holiday to Spain, wrote to both Marthe and Bonnard, then returned to Paris and killed herself there in a hotel. It is thought by some that she died in the bath.* Shortly after that, in 1925, Bonnard and Marthe were married. In that year too, he began to paint the famous series of images of the woman in the bath that he continued for another twenty years. Unlike many of his other nude paintings, there is no obvious precursor to this pose in

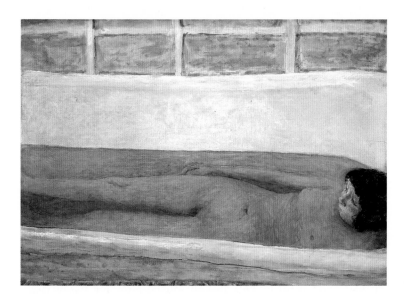

'The bath' by Pierre Bonnard (1925)

*For instance, see *Nudes and landscapes* by Sasha Newman.[19] It appears to be denied, however, by a letter in 1993 from Bonnard's great-nephew Michel Terrasse to Belinda Thomson.[20] Michel Terrasse has published two books on Bonnard.

classical sculpture or in the paintings of colleagues. Though the nude in the bath is physically like Marthe, who was then 56 years old and often bathing, most commentators agree that these are certainly portraits of a woman who was very much younger, and seems to remain young throughout the series. Is this Bonnard's memory of the young Marthe, or, in their morgue-like stillness, of Renée, or have the images of two women merged?

It is not public knowledge what the relationship between these three was. What is clear is that Renée's death (coming just after the deaths of his brother-in-law Claude Terrasse and his sister, and Bonnard's own serious pneumonia) 'deeply distressed [Bonnard]; he never parted with some of the works she had inspired, and insisted on including them unobtrusively in his exhibition cata- logues and in anything written on his painting'.* He reworked parts of the *Young women in the garden*, the portrait of Renée, after Marthe's death in 1942.

This description of my response to this painting is not a claim about history: I am not an art historian. There is much that prob- ably will never be known about Bonnard's private life, and other interpretations of *The open window* could be offered. But what I want to give is an account of my reaction, how distress in a secre- tive artist might have transmitted itself to an observer who, at the time, knew nothing about the possibility of such distress. How could this interpretation have come about? What are the cues or clues?

One was clearly the subject matter. Bonnard painted many interiors, and many of his paintings show windows and doors, with views beyond. This painting is one of the few where the view is central *and* the window is open. The trees are painted much more clearly than the room; although this painter often makes the marginal objects more blurred and diverts attention from them, the focus of the painting is on the wilderness of trees in the garden. To me at the time, *The open window* was a picture about a tragic choice for Bonnard, a man in midlife, between a woman he had lived with, looked at, and looked after for many years,

---

*From a written communication from Antoine Terrasse, one of Bonnard's other great-nephews, who wrote an authoritative monograph on his great uncle and has made other major contributions to the bibliography on Bonnard, including extracts from the painter's diaries.

reclusive, inside, stifling; and a younger, more exciting, and freer love in the freshness of nature. Separating these hung the guillotine of decision.

The language of being a patient

Bonnard was 54 when he painted this picture. This is a vulnerable period for relationships, as evidenced by the problems brought week after week to GP surgeries and counselling agencies by people at this time of life. But if my interpretation is at all near the mark, Bonnard had little he could do with this distress, no outlet other than his work. This was not a story which could be openly told, other than through the medium which he habitually used, that of paint and colour. Was I misreading the 'text' of this painting? When Rembrandt, for instance, painted his amazing series of self portraits, modern commentators remind us that, moving self-revelations as they may be to us, they were not primarily intended this way and were often to demonstrate his prowess.[21]

Such contrasts in approach and interpretation are part of the wonder of looking at art from another age. It is as if we may outline our own sensibilities against the light of great art from times past. What we may then read in that art, or what that artist may make us read in ourselves, may be one of the marks of greatness in that work – the 'tingle' factor, as some would have it now. As we look or read, however, we must beware of foisting our current standards or sensibility upon that artist. My reaction to Bonnard was that of a twentieth century doctor, and that reaction required (and received) some considerable attention and thought. But when all is said and done, whether the surmises about the long-term effects of Renée's death on his subsequent work are correct, it would take a lot to persuade me that in *The open window* he was not communicating something of his intense distress about what must have been a terrible dilemma.

That this could come across so loudly across three quarters of a century to someone not a professional artist may bear witness to the intensity of the feeling that is conveyed through that painting. But did Bonnard know what he was doing? Renée's drawn portrait is in those trees, so it suggests that at some psychological level he did: but that probably at another level, these feelings were hard for him to express. When later she died at her own hand, as we would expect, whatever their real relationship, he was deeply distressed, and remained so. Although he wrote diaries, however, we find no word about it there.* He recorded mostly aphorisms or just the ordinary things which were important to his work – the weather, the light.[22] As an artist, he communicated largely through his painting. For those who are not gifted artists, this form of communication may not be available. Others may not be able to communicate through words, or may not yet have the words needed to express their feelings or distress.

Helping patients to find an outlet for distress

During a recent evening surgery a young couple came to see me as an emergency, with a newborn girl baby and a very active toddler. The emergency was the older boy. Since the birth of the baby, he was pissing everywhere. 'And tonight,' said the desperate mum, 'he pissed on the baby.' I could not help smiling. 'You laugh, doctor?' she exploded. 'But she's the most precious thing in the world … Oh my God, what have I said?' Through tears and hugs this little family suddenly realised what their toddler had been trying to say to them – that he mattered, that they had forgotten him in their excitement about the new baby, that he had been 'passed' over, 'eliminated', as it were, from the centre of their attention.

The thought is sophisticated, the symbolism both complex and stark: but the child had no other way of expressing it. He was lucky, because his parents were part of a new way of thinking which looked for emotional communication and understood how important their love was for him. His mother noticed my smile: and I sometimes think that had I been more 'professional' and kept a straight face, or had she not taken offence at my expression, that family would still be involved in weekly psychotherapy, or the child attending some paediatric urology service.

These parents were alert and attentive to their children's needs, but I do not think the good or immediate outcome we shared that evening would have easily occurred in the 1970s or before. There

---

*There remains the possibility that more will come to light. There was a legal battle over his estate, and some writings which were handed over then seem not yet to have been published.

has been a change over my professional lifetime in the way people think about family relationships and communication, about how they see their bodies, and about what they consider relevant and appropriate to bring to professional attention. Whether professionals are behind or ahead of the mainstream is difficult to say, but for me and other colleagues the frustration in the 1970s of trying to help patients whom we met to 'connect' with their inner selves has led some doctors to adopt a different approach in general practice. We hear the language of the patient's complaint and, as GPs, we learn to listen to other things as well, to link change and loss and distress to a discourse which before was confined to entirely physical sensations.

What is your body trying to tell you?

But how real is this? Is this medical paternalism in a new and very insidious form? Am I like a latter-day critic making false attributions to a Rembrandt or Bonnard? Does this process represent something that really exists? Could the body be speaking to the individual, the self who lives in that body, through symptoms, because that individual is not aware of, or refusing to listen to, other messages from the body? People vary, times change: but I have no doubt that it often requires an outsider to point out connections between symptoms and other facets of a person's life because true self-consciousness is so hard.

Pierre Bonnard could not express his distress except in paint. The toddler could not get through to his mother the desperation he felt. Some people perhaps cannot hear what their bodies are trying to tell them. Where there is no change and the trouble continues, it is as if symptoms may be the only way in which one part of the individual may communicate with another. Symptoms become a language in themselves. So the question could be put in a consultation, 'What is your body trying to tell you?'

I still remember one of the first times that I used that phrase, on a Saturday morning in the late 1970s when a woman came in with sudden new upper abdominal pain so severe that initially I thought I should admit her at once to hospital. But when I had asked her, 'What is your body trying to tell you?' she burst into tears and told me how she could not stand any longer going out with her older boyfriend, who would make no moves to consolidate their relationship. Once she had said this to me, the pain began gradually to resolve.

Upper abdominal pain as a sign of emotional distress is not a new idea: the ancient Greeks were aware of sensations here, and thought the stomach was the seat of the emotions. The Greek word 'phrēn' was associated with thinking and emotion and is left in our own medical language bizarrely divided between the connections to the mind (as in 'schizophrenia') and its physical site in the name of the nerve to the diaphragm (the 'phrenic nerve'). That Saturday patient was obviously distressed. Without the encouragement I had received from my teachers in general practice to explore more broadly, I would probably have, incorrectly, assumed her distress was due to the pain, and might not have discovered that the pain was, in fact, due to her distress.*

Talking and being listened to

For some reason our emotional life is a part of ourselves that all of us, doctors and patients, face up to with difficulty, with many people continuing to deny its relevance in medicine. Not everyone will be convinced by the idea of two parts (or more) of an individual's consciousness, or of two or multiple selves, or of hidden meaning in the symptoms or actions of any individual. Modern medical thinking has found some further insight through the concept of narrative in illness.[23] Though sometimes the patient simply has a story to tell, and may or may not be able to tell it or have it listened to, narrative medicine also hears a deeper story, told through the patient's aims, desires, fears, expectations and reactions.

Sometimes, different consultations are like fragments of stories, half interrupted elements, which need to be put together.[24] The fragments may be detected in dreams, but may also tell their story through body reactions. Such narratives may not hang together well, or be understood in the short term. They may need longer-term or deeper work, with professional help in psychotherapy: or people may piece them together for themselves through their own

---

*This was the sort of approach opened up to me by John McEwan and Raymond Pietroni during my training at Princess Street in the Elephant and Castle.

conversations or writing. Identifying difficulties and discontinuities is one thing, but changing them is quite another. Proving that talking treatments are better than other approaches, like letting things ride or repressing feelings, is difficult. I believe they usually are, and that this will eventually be clearly proved. I believe counselling, available now at most general practices in south London, is a vital part of our primary care service. But the point I wish to make here is this: that having begun to understand something of this new language, people will want to learn it for themselves, to learn to listen to it, to speak it. People want to talk about their inner lives, and talk to someone who will listen. But what if no one wants to listen, or has time to hear?

Suffering and the self

There are many things of course that people do not care to talk about. An interesting example is the discussion of impending death. In more religious times, it was customary to prepare oneself openly for death. In the nineteenth century, doctors described discussing a poor prognosis quite frankly and straightforwardly with patients.[25] If people were going to die, doctors told them they were, and they seemed to be grateful for this openness. By the time I had begun to practise, such discussions were extremely uncommon. When I was training, I seldom heard the doctors I accompanied in my work discuss dying. It was as if this subject had become taboo: with the coming of antibiotics and improving public health and a dramatic reduction in the deaths of children and young adults, the topic seems to have been banished from the wards. In general practice, although fear of dying hovered over many consultations, it had become difficult to discuss this threat openly. In its place, as has been seen, symptoms loomed large. This anxiety about discussing death remains widespread.

In parallel, some observers have seen a shift in how people in Western society would describe the best in life, their highest aims. The philosopher Charles Taylor has pointed out in his study of modern selfhood that when modern society searches for the good it looks towards ordinary life – work, leisure, sexual fulfilments, friendships, family. As well as 'modern inwardness', he sees 'the affirmation of ordinary life' as being key to our identity. Part of this, in common with other higher civilisations, is the importance we put on avoiding suffering.[26] This links with modern experience. An individual's experience of death nowadays is more likely to be that of an elderly relative whose quality of life has sunk very low, or of someone in midlife struggling and failing to control the advance of a cancer. Sudden unexpected deaths are news. It is not life, but a life that's worth living, that is of most concern. Death's place at the top of the league of things we openly discuss as wanting to avoid has been taken by irremediable pain, or other types of suffering which devastate and prevent people from getting on with their lives. Modern secular society may see death as a distant final objective event, but fears suffering as a prevalent and subjective state. It is one which can destroy life by destroying the enjoyment of life.

This brings an old problem of medicine back to centre stage. What is subjective may be very hard to define, and impossible to measure. It is difficult for a clinician to assess a patient's pain, for instance, or to measure it outside the laboratory, without using words. The words that are used may be shared but have different values, depending on the speaker. This problem is built into the centre of medical practice. In most languages, certainly in Europe, the words for illness and disease are, like their counterparts in English, derived from subjective words or ideas: being 'ill', 'unwell', not at 'ease' are all largely associated with inner thoughts, not external signs.[27] So neither patient or professional is let off the hook. Though there may be no objective sign of a disease, the presence of distress or pain is another thing. To explain suffering we must all listen to and pay attention to the individual's account of what is going on.

The need to share in order to heal

Through modern media, our society has been introduced to accounts of tragic events as perhaps never before. But even the accounts of the worst of these sometimes hold a paradox. Primo Levi, a Holocaust survivor writing about the terrible events at Auschwitz, describes drifting off to sleep in his shared bunk. He dreams of being at home in Italy, talking to his sister and her friends. He is telling them about the horrors of the camp, and what he is going through. Gradually, they begin to talk amongst themselves, and take no notice of him or what he is saying. He wakes up in a cold sweat of rejection. When he wakes he realises he keeps on dreaming this dream. He then discovers from talking to other Italian Jews in the camp that they too are dreaming this, the dream of the unlistened-to story.[28] Something new has happened here. Under threat of extermination, the impending death of the person is hidden by something apparently bigger perhaps because nearer: the realisation that as he suffers, no-one is listening to his account of his suffering.

This seems to me to be one of the keys to modern sensibility, part of the difference, as it were, between what I observed in my surgery in the 1970s and what I see today. To suffer is terrible, but to be unable to talk about it to someone who will give that talk proper attention is very much worse. Given our basic natures, it seems that a toddler unattended by his mother or a person whose lover has died has always felt distress, certainly in the recent years of mankind's history. It also seems likely, however, that the cultural expression of such distress or the value given to it will have varied greatly; that even within the same language the words used, and the attention and meaning given to those words, will have altered over time.

In my lifetime I believe I have seen a shift in the way 'distress talk' is handled in the society in which I have lived. Suffering seems to have become not just associated with a *feeling* of distress as with the inability to *share* that feeling with an appropriate person as well. Even if that is taking an extreme view, there is no doubt that pain and its related symptoms remind people of their 'aloneness' like few other things can do. For most of us, happiness is increased by sharing, either directly with others, or with our own memories of other people, or expectations across time. When we suffer, even if others are suffering similarly, our suffering is unique, and ours alone.

Coping with suffering, healing its effects, some would now say, needs a return to sharing. Someone needs to pay attention, to validate the experience, to 'be there' to listen and to share the burden. When Diana died, the world was amazed as the UK, known (amongst other things) for emotional restraint, went wild with grief. Even subtracting the power of the media to drum up crowd hysteria about the premature death of a beautiful public figure, this outpouring of grief carried for me a powerful message. When I spoke to patients or colleagues, they reported similar interpretations of this phenomena. To the grieving public, Diana represented someone who was prepared to listen, to show she cared by touching the apparently untouchable. In spite of her own all too obvious flaws, her own needs included her need to talk about these very needs and, in that respect at least, people felt she was 'one of us'.

Conclusion

I have suggested that the medical landscape has changed significantly over the last fifty years, with people who visit a professional in health care now expecting to be involved in the decision-making. They expect to be a part, and a key part, of the partnership or team that is providing the care. When that relationship, between patient and professional, goes wrong, the source of the problem may be found in the failure of one or both parties to understand themselves, often in the most basic sense of the feelings, fears or expectations they bring to that encounter. It is now considered highly desirable in our society for patients to learn to make sense of symptoms and gain meaning from their experiences through a clinical encounter, and in the context of health care, for a patient not to be listened *to* is becoming increasingly intolerable. People want to be able to explore their fears or bad experiences, to try to make sense of them. When they are not allowed to, this seems like a real deprivation, a yet further increase in suffering. Whether I am right about the interpretation I give of a picture matters not a jot. But if I am even half right about what our society now needs, how it sees suffering, and about the response it requires, then both the organisers and receivers of health care have a lot of hard thinking to do.

References

1 Editor's introduction to Hume D, Beauchamp T (ed). *An essay concerning the principles of morals*. Oxford: Oxford University Press, 1998.
2 See, for instance, Pinker S. *The blank slate*. London: Penguin Books, 2002.

3   See 'As, rule of' in Boyd K, Higgs R, Pinching A (eds), *The new dictionary of medical ethics*. London: BMJ Books, 1997.

4   Hennessy P. *Never again: Britain 1945–51*. London: Jonathan Cape, 1992.

5   Heron A (ed). *Towards a Quaker view of sex: an essay by a group of friends*. London: Friends Home Service Committee, 1963.

6   Robinson J. *Honest to God*. London: SCM Press, 1963.

7   Bowlby J. *Attachment and loss*. London: Hogarth Press, 1969.

8   Higgs R. An example of intermediate care: the new Lambeth Community Care Centre. *BMJ* 1985;**291**:1395–7.

9   Described in a series of articles in the *Architects Journal* special issue of 16th October 1985, 42 vol 182.

10 Higgs R. Unemployment in my practice. *BMJ* 1981;**283**:532.

11 See Curran and Higgs 'Setting up a counsellor in primary care' in Corney R, Jenkins R (eds). *Counselling in general practice*. London: Routledge, 1992.

12 Mayou R, Bass C, Sharpe M (eds). *Treatment of functional somatic symptoms*. Oxford: Oxford University Press, 1995.

13 Skynner R. *One flesh: separate persons*. London: Constable, 1976.

14 Higgs R. *Psychosocial problems: a workbook for general practice 1*. Minneapolis, MN: Modern Medicine Publications, 1983.

15 Higgs R, 'Psychological issues in general practice'. In: Stephenson A (ed). *A textbook of general practice*. London: Arnold, 1998.

16 Balint M. *The doctor, his patient and the illness*. London: Pitman Medical, 1964.

17 O'Dowd TC. Five years of heartsink patients in general practice. *BMJ* 1988;**297**(6647):528–30.

18 Whitfield S. *Bonnard*. London: Tate Gallery Publishing, 1998.

19 Newman S, 'Nudes and landscapes'. In: *Bonnard: the graphic work*. New York: The Metropolitan Museum of Art, 1989.

20 Terrasse M, 'Pierre Bonnard: private life, public reputation'. In: *Bonnard at Les Bosquet*. London: The South Bank Centre, 1994.

21 van de Wetering E, 'The multiple function of Rembrandt's self-portraits'. In: White C, Buvelot Q (eds). *Rembrandt by himself*. London: National Gallery Publications, 1999.

22 A selection of entries were published with notes by Antoine Terrasse in: *Bonnard*. Paris: Centre Georges Pompidou, 1984.

23 For instance see Brody H. *Stories of sickness*. New Haven, CT: Yale University Press, 1987 and Greenhalgh T, Hurwitz B (eds). *Narrative based medicine*. London: BMJ Books, 1998.

24 See Holmes J, 'Narrative Psychotherapy'. In: Greenhalgh T and Hurwitz B (eds). *Narrative based medicine*. London: BMJ Books, 1998.

25 A wonderful example is the account of the death of Nelson given by his physician Dr William Beatty, in Lewis J (ed). *The mammoth book of how it happened*. London: Robinson Publishing, 1998.

26 Taylor C. *Sources of the self: the making of the modern identity*. Cambridge: Cambridge University Press, 1989.

27 Wolff H. *Philosophy of medicine*. Oxford: Blackwell, 1990.

28 Levi P. *If this is a man*. London: Sphere, 1987.

Epilogue

KENNETH CALMAN

An epilogue is an addition at the end of a book. It might also be seen as the last word. But in a subject like this it cannot, and should not, be the last word. To paraphrase Churchill, this is not the end, but the end of the beginning.

The history of the connections between the arts and health is very long, stretching back into the mists of time. However, it is only in the last two decades that the discipline, or more properly the range of disciplines, of the arts in health has cohered and developed a character and vision of its own.

A danger, however, is the temptation to put the 'arts and health' in a box, with artificial boundaries created by those leading the projects taking place across the country. Part of the excitement of this whole area is that the boundaries keep shifting. New and different ways in which the arts and humanities might play a role in improving health become apparent all the time. The arts in health field should, I believe, be inclusive, not exclusive, and all those who have an interest in contributing should be able to do so.

The title of this book, 'The healing environment', sets the tone. The chapters examine in various ways the role that a range of different arts and humanities can play in assisting healing. The word 'healing' is itself important, deriving as it does from 'wholeness'; a much wider and comprehensive term than 'cure'. There is a distinction between illness and wholeness; people can be physically unwell and still be 'whole', and while cure may not be possible in all instances, healing can occur.

Five factors can be seen to play a key part in determining health and well-being. Firstly, advances in our understanding of genetic and biological factors offer the promise of improvements in health. The second factor is the formal health services, who do a great job of sorting out problems once they have occurred. How and where these health services are delivered can matter a great deal to patients and their families. For example, the setting of health care – buildings, colours, fabrics, music – can do much to improve well-being and reduce anxiety. This is well demonstrated in the book.

Then there are social and economic factors such as employment, poverty, housing, deprivation and family. These can have a significant impact on health, and all can be improved by the arts. The arts have an important role in improving the health of the community: public art, music and theatre can all influence the quality of life of a whole community. The fourth factor that influences health is lifestyle, which includes our attitude to alcohol, drugs, and diet. Music and dance can play a significant role in changing lifestyle and improving health.

The final factor affecting health and well-being is the physical environment, including the built environment in which we live and work. The role of architecture in influencing our emotions has sometimes been forgotten both in health care and in society in general. Buildings can have a major impact on health and on how we feel, and our quality of life can be significantly affected by the physical environment we inhabit.

This leads to the heart of this book for me: the whole topic of quality of life. Quality of life is difficult to define, and is a concept which varies from individual to individual. Aspirations for an improved quality of life represent the gap between what we are and our expectations. The quality of life an individual aspires to is therefore the difference between what is and what might be.[1] The arts in all their many forms can help narrow the gap, improving the quality of life by providing something extra.

Implicit in this definition is the acknowledgment that as we are all individuals, not all of us will be influenced by the same things, whether they fall into the categories of music, the visual arts or literature. Even within these broad areas there will be differences and health service providers should not expect their personal preferences to be taken up by everyone. Some people like jazz and others classical music. We cannot impose our values. In the words of Mark Twain, 'If your only tool is a hammer, all your problems will be nails'.

This book argues that the arts can therefore create the environment in which healing and an improved quality of life can occur. But is this really so? Is well-being improved by listening to music, or reading a poem, or seeing a play? What is the evidence? Fortunately the intuitive feelings of many people working in the field are now beginning to be supported by such evidence, some of which is well set out in this book. My own reading suggests that blood pressure can be lowered, pre-operative anxiety reduced, and pain control improved by the use of humour.[2] Examining things closely, studying them, analysing them, however, can take away from the sheer joy of listening and looking. Jokes become meaningless if you have to explain them. But it is clear that if the arts are to be used to improve the service provided to patients and the public then this kind of research is essential. We owe it to our patients to understand these mechanisms because this curiosity is an important part of improving the care we provide.

Nor must doctors, or others in health care, allow themselves to become hidebound. The increasing use of new media – such as the Internet and virtual reality – and the new creative arts, present opportunities to appeal to different groups of users. In a play by Aristophanes, a character is asked, 'What do you want a poet for?' The reply is, 'To save the city of course'. We might ask the same question of the new creative arts and get the same answer.

There is another theme running through this book, and that is of the use of stories. The stories in *The healing environment* may be personal or about others. They are all remarkably powerful. Quotations by patients and staff bring the issues to life and add a dimension which is vibrant and real. Human beings learn through stories and remember them; they create the environment within which it is possible to learn from the experiences of others. These stories are used to communicate with and benefit others. Doctors should not be afraid to share stories, but should recognise that they are part of a wider range of literature and need to be interpreted accordingly.

The whole area of the arts and health has come a long way. Its role is now being discussed by patients, clinicians, managers and policy makers. Several groups are engaged in research into the effectiveness of arts-related interventions. The range of project work being undertaken across the UK is astonishing, and we can all benefit from the lessons being learnt. A personal story may illustrate this. Several years ago I visited a newly-built care centre for those with learning difficulties. It was beautifully constructed with a wide range of tactile and visual experiences. One of these was the replacement of down pipes from the roof gutters by chains, so that as the rain fell it cascaded down the chains, creating a beautiful effect. Afterwards, I moved into a house in which one of the down pipes was missing and replaced it with a chain instead of a pipe. Now I am able to experience for myself the calming effect of the falling water. A lesson passed on.

The evidence base for the valuable contribution the arts and humanities can make to health and well-being is growing. Patients are already feeling the difference their own efforts and those of others have made. Through an active involvement patients can, as they surely must, become connected with and part of the health care process. Now is the time to build on all of these experiences, and so this epilogue is really a prologue for the next book, and for the series of initiatives which are now needed to take things even further.

References

1   Calman KC. Quality of life in cancer patients: an hypothesis. *J Medical Ethics* 1984;**10**:124-7.
2   Calman KC. *A study of story telling, humour and learning in medicine.* London: HMSO, 2000.

Further reading

This reading list has been compiled from the suggestions of contributors with the intention of sharing with readers some works they have found valuable. It is by no means exhaustive.

Medical humanities and narrative-based medicine

Evans M, Finlay I. *Medical humanities*. London: BMJ Books, 2001.

Greenhalgh P, Hurwitz B. *Narrative based medicine*. London: BMJ Books, 1998.

Hunsaker Hawkins A, Chandler McIntyre M (eds). *Teaching literature and medicine*. New York: Modern Language Association, 2000.

Kirklin D, Richardson R (eds). *Medical humanities: a practical introduction*. London: Royal College of Physicians, 2001.

Launer J, *Narrative-based primary care: a practical guide*. Abingdon: Radcliffe Medical Press, 2002.

Morley D (ed). *The gift: new writing for the NHS*. Exeter: Stride Publications, 2002.

Patient-centred care

Berger J, Mohr J. *A fortunate man*. London: Royal College of General Practitioners, 2003.

Campbell A, Higgs R. *In that case*. London: Darton Longman and Todd, 1982.

Casement P. *On learning from the patient*. London: Routledge, 1985.

Miller A. *The drama of being a child*. London: Virago, 1987.

Neighbour R. *The inner consultation*. Reading: Petroc Press, 1987.

Nussbaum M. *The fragility of goodness*. Cambridge: Cambridge University Press, 2001.

MacDonald G, O'Hara K. *Ten elements of mental health, its promotion and demotion: implications for practice*. Glasgow: Society of Health Education and Health Promotion Specialists, 1998.

Rogers C. *Client centred therapy*. London: Constable and Robinson, 1976.

Looking at art

Armstrong J. *The intimate philosophy of art*. London: Penguin, 2000.

Ball P. *Bright earth, art and the invention of colour*. New York: Farrar, Straus and Giroux, 2001.

Bell J. *What is painting?* London: Thames and Hudson, 1999.

Berger J. *Ways of seeing*. London: Penguin, 1990.

Birren F. *The symbolism of colour*. New York: Carol Publishing, 1988.

Dittrich L (ed). *Ten years of medicine and the arts*. Washington, DC: American Association of Medical Colleges, 2001.

Gaskell I. *Vermeer's wager: speculations on art history, theory and art museums (Essays in Art and Culture)*. London: Reaktion, 2001.

Gombrich EH. *The story of art*. London: Phaidon Press, 1995.

Gregory RL. *Eye and brain: the psychology of seeing*. Oxford: Oxford University Press, 1997.

Kandinsky W. *Concerning the spiritual in art*. New York: Dover Publications, 1977.

Lamb T, Bourriau J (eds). *Colour, art and science*. Cambridge: Cambridge University Press, 1995.

Lancaster M. *Colourscape*: New York: Wiley Academy, 1996.

Langmuir E. *The National Gallery companion guide*. London: National Gallery Publications, 1999.

Murray L, Howard B. *Angels and monsters: a child's view of cancer*. Atlanta, GA: American Cancer Society, 2002.

Osbourne R. *Lights and pigments, colour principles for artists*. London: John Murray, 1980.

Petrone M. *The emotional cancer journey*. London: MAP Foundation, 2003.

Petrone M. *Touching the rainbow: pictures and words by people affected* by *cancer*. Brighton: MAP Foundation, 2003.

Porter T, Mikellides B. *Colour for architecture*. London: Studio Vista, 1976.

Snunit M. *The soul bird*. London: Constable and Robinson, 1998.

Southgate MT. *The art of JAMA vol 1*. Chicago: AMA Press, 1997.

Southgate MT. The art of JAMA vol 2. Chicago: AMA Press, 2001.

Art, architecture and design in therapeutic settings

Arts Council of England. *Arts in healthcare directory*. London: Arts Council of England, 2002.

Baron JH. Art in hospitals: the Fitzpatrick Lecture 1994. *J R Coll Physicians Lond* 1995;**29**:131–144.

Dilani A. Design and health: the therapeutic benefits of design. Stockholm: AB Svensk Byggtjänst, 2001.

Friedrich MJ. *The arts of healing.* 1999;**281**(19):1779–81.

Gardner N, 'The art of good health: using visual arts in healthcare'. In: Holmes S (ed). *Improving the patient experience.* London: Stationery Office Books/ NHS Estates, 2002.

Haldane D, Loppert S (eds). *The arts in healthcare: learning from experience.* London: King's Fund, 1999.

Lawson B, Phiri M, Wells-Thorpe J. The architectural healthcare environment and its effects on patient health outcomes. London: NHS Estates/ The Stationery Office, 2003.

Medical Architecture Research Unit. *Innovative environments for rehabilitation.* London: South Bank University, 1999.

The Nuffield Trust. *Building a 2020 vision: future healthcare environments.* London: The Stationery Office, 2001.

Poetry therapy and creative writing

Bly R, Hillman J, Meade M (eds). *The rag and bone shop of the heart.* London: HarperCollins: 1993.

Bolton G. *Reflective practice: writing and professional development.* London: Paul Chapman Publishing, 2001.

Campo R. *The healing art: a doctor's black bag of poetry.* New York: WW Norton, 2003.

Coulehan J, Belli A (eds). *Blood and bone: poems by physicians.* Iowa City, IA: University of Iowa Press, 1998.

Davis C, Scaefer J (eds).*Between the heartbeats: poems and prose by nurses.* Iowa City, IA: University of Iowa Press, 1995.

Davis C, Scaefer J (eds). *Intensive care: more poetry and prose by nurses.* Iowa City, IA: University of Iowa Press, 2003.

Fox J. *Finding what you didn't lose: expressing your truth and creativity through poem-making.* New York: Tarcher Putnam, 1995.

Fox J. *Poetic medicine: the healing art of poem-making.* New York: Tarcher Putnam, 1997.

Hynes A, Hynes-Berry M. *Biblio-poetry therapy: the interactive process. A handbook.* St Cloud, MN: North Star Press, 1986.

Kelley A. *The poetry remedy.* Penzance: Hypatia Trust & Patten Press, 1999.

Sewell M (ed). *Cries of the spirit.* Boston, MA: Houghton Mifflin, 1991.

Waldman MR (ed). *Healer: dancing with the healing spirit.* New York: Jeremy P Tarcher/GP Putnam, 2003.

Weisberger LL, Chavis GG (eds). *The healing fountain: poetry therapy for life's journey.* St Cloud, MN: North Star Press, 2003.

Loss

Hazzard A, Weston J, Gutterres C. After a child's death: factors related to parental bereavement. *J Dev Behav Pediatr* 1992;**13**(1):24–30.

Klein HK. *Gili's book: a journey into bereavement for parents and counsellors*. New York: Teacher's College Press, 1998.

Rando T. Bereaved parents: particular difficulties, unique factors, and treatment issues. *Soc Work* 1985;**30**(1):19–23.

Rowe M. Metamorphosis: defending the human. *Lit Med* 2002;**21**(2): 264–80

Rowe M. *The book of Jesse: a story of youth, illness, and medicine*. Washington, DC: Francis Press, 2002.

Useful websites and databases

Centre for Medical Humanities
www.pcps.ucl.ac.uk/cmh

UCL Medical Humanities Resource Database
www.mhrd.ucl.ac.uk

National Gallery (includes information on every painting in the collection)
www.nationalgallery.org.uk

The National Network for Arts in Healthcare (United Kingdom)
www.nnah.org.uk

The National Association for Poetry Therapy (United States)
www.poetrytherapy.org

The Association for Literary Arts in Personal Development
www.lapidus.org.uk

John Fox's website about poetry therapy
www.poeticmedicine.com

The Mind Arts Project in Stockport
www.mindartsproject.co.uk

The MAP Foundation
www.mapfoundation.org

Copyright acknowledgements

Cover
'Anam cara' by Michele Petrone
reproduced by permission of the artist.

Chapter 2
All images reproduced by permission
of Bob Curtis Photography, Brighton.

Chapter 3
Nineteenth century and modern
images of the Royal London Hospital
outpatients' department reproduced
by permission of the Royal London
Hospital Archives. Aerial view of the
old St Thomas's Hospital reproduced
by permission of the Wellcome
Library, London.

Chapter 4
All images reproduced by permission
of the National Gallery, London,
except 'The garden enclosed'
which is copyright the Tate, London
2003 and reproduced with
permission of the trustees of
the David Jones Estate.

Chapter 5
All images reproduced courtesy of
Chelsea and Westminster Hospital
Arts.

Chapter 6
All images reproduced by permission
of the author.

Chapter 7
All images reproduced by permission
of the Mind Arts Project in Stockport.

Chapter 8
'Release (Swingeing London III)'
© Richard Hamilton 2003. All rights
reserved, DACS. Stills from the film of
Trainspotting reproduced by
permission of FilmFour.
Photographer: Liam Langman.

Chapter 9
'Shadow' by Michele Petrone
reproduced by permission of the
artist.

Chapter 10
All images reproduced by permission
of the author.

Chapter 11
'Esparragal' reproduced by permission
of Maxine Relton. The poems
'Bendición', 'One morning', 'The
remedies', 'Lunch with a pathologist'
and 'Mary Rivers' are reproduced by
permission of their authors. 'At
Blackwater Pond' © 1978 by Mary
Oliver. Used with permission of The
Molly Malone Cook Literary Agency.

Chapter 12
'The open window' by Pierre Bonnard
reproduced by permission of the
Phillips Collection, Washington DC.
'The bath' by Pierre Bonnard.
© ADAGP, Paris and DACS, London
2003.

Index

A more detailed index can be found on the Royal College of Physicians website:
www.rcplondon.ac.uk/pubs/healingenv.pdf